The Madness Within Us

The Madness Within Us

Schizophrenia as a Neuronal Process

Robert Freedman

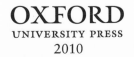

OXFORD

UNIVERSITY PRESS

2010

OXFORD
UNIVERSITY PRESS

Oxford University Press, Inc., publishes works that further
Oxford University's objective of excellence
in research, scholarship, and education.

Oxford   New York
Auckland   Cape Town   Dar es Salaam   Hong Kong   Karachi
Kuala Lumpur   Madrid   Melbourne   Mexico City   Nairobi
New Delhi   Shanghai   Taipei   Toronto

With offices in
Argentina   Austria   Brazil   Chile   Czech Republic   France   Greece
Guatemala   Hungary   Italy   Japan   Poland   Portugal   Singapore
South Korea   Switzerland   Thailand   Turkey   Ukraine   Vietnam

Published by Oxford University Press, Inc.
198 Madison Avenue, New York, New York 10016

www.oup.com

Oxford is a registered trademark of Oxford University Press, Inc.

Library of Congress Cataloging-in-Publication Data

Freedman, Robert, 1946–
The madness within us : schizophrenia as a neuronal
process / Robert Freedman.
p.   ;   cm.
Includes bibliographical references.
ISBN-13: 978-0-19-530747-4 (alk. paper)
ISBN-10: 0-19-530747-X (alk. paper)
1. Schizophrenia. 2. Neuropsychiatry. I. Title.
[DNLM: 1. Schizophrenic Psychology. 2. Brain—physiopathology.
3. Brain Chemistry. 4. Models, Neurological. 5. Nerve Degeneration.
6. Schizophrenia—etiology. WM 203 F853m 2009]
RC514.F695 2009
616.89′8—dc22
2009009500

9 8 7 6 5 4 3 2 1

Printed in the United States of America on acid-free paper

Acknowledgments

I am grateful to my patients who have worked patiently with me while I tried to understand and treat them to the best of my ability.

My teachers Barry Hoffer and the late Jarl Dyrud taught me neurobiology and how to listen to people who were trying to teach me something.

My colleagues, Sherry Leonard, Randy Ross, Lawrence Adler, Lars Olson, Homer Olsen, Ann Olincy, Herbert Nagamoto, Paula Bickford, Christine Miller, Karen Stevens, Cathy Adams, Allan Collins, William Byerley, William Kem, Pablo Gejman, David Braff, Josette Harris, Laura Martin, Merilyne Waldo, Yiping Du, and Jason Tregellas have taught me wonderful things about the science and practice of psychiatry. Roberta Payne, Ph.D., gave me moral support and Elaine Steffen helped me with the manuscript. Joan Bossert was a wonderfully patient editor.

My work has been supported by gifts from Jerome H. Kern and Mary Rossick Kern, John and Janet Albers, Richard Saunders, and Sam and Dr. Nancy Gary, and research grants from the National Institute of Mental Health, the Department of Veterans Affairs, NARSAD, and the Stanley Foundation.

My wife Sari made sure that I never gave up my dreams. She and my children, Aaron, Jason, and Andrew, and my parents have unfailingly supported all that I have wanted to do.

Contents

Preface

This book is intended to introduce readers to schizophrenia as an illness of the human mind and the brain. People who develop this illness are treated with drugs that are intended to moderate the effects of the illness on how their brain works and with psychotherapy that is intended to guide their personal recovery. We will discuss both in this book, because both are critical aspects of their treatment. We will follow two patients over the course of the book, Paul and Rachel. Both are disguised composites of patients whom I have had the privilege of working with and learning from over the past decades.

The book is not directed to my many colleagues who conduct research into the causes and treatments of schizophrenia. They would recognize, as do I, that there are many stories to tell about the neurobiology of schizophrenia. To try to tell them all, giving each its proper weight, would require many volumes. Similarly, the clinical vignettes are not intended to teach my clinical colleagues about the treatment of schizophrenia. Those who treat schizophrenia will recognize that people who have this illness present a wealth of challenges that are often far more overwhelming than those summarized in the vignettes about Rachel and Paul.

In this book, I attempt to bridge a gap between the understanding of schizophrenia as a problem in the activity of nerve cells and the human experience of having schizophrenia. A dichotomy between the body and mind is often held to be one of the failings of Western philosophy, generally attributed to Descartes, who first posed this dualism as a problem and then failed to find a solution beyond faith. Schizophrenia is the most uniquely human of all mental disorders, because its most characteristic symptom is disordered thinking. It is also one of the most intensively researched disorders at the neurobiological level. It has long occurred to me that to consider schizophrenia from both perspectives simultaneously would illuminate how specific neuronal mechanisms are involved in the process of thinking.

Many have proposed that a definitive understanding of mind–brain interactions is impossible, but these authors have not considered an illness like schizophrenia as a focal point of their investigation. Throughout the history of medicine, diseases have revealed mechanisms that were otherwise imperceptible in normal persons. The exquisite regulation of glucose metabolism is an example of a mechanism that only revealed itself in the problems of diabetic individuals. However, it also fair to say that this book is not a rigorous philosophical or scientific treatise, because there are many philosophical and scientific issues that it does not address.[1]

Instead, I have made this a personal book about the investigations of my research group into one of the neuronal dysfunctions found in schizophrenia, a defect in sensory gating, and the experiences of patients with whom I have worked. The goal was not a definitive solution, because one does not yet exist, but rather to tell what we have learned to future generations of medical and graduate students and other interested people who might expand the understanding of schizophrenia with their own investigations and clinical experiences. I also hope that the book will be helpful to families and individuals who are dealing with mental illness and want to understand how these illnesses happen. Therefore, although there is much technical material, I have tried to make the explanations as simple as possible to allow the book to be accessible to those who are just becoming interested in how the brain works. Notes are provided for those who want to read about the same material from the research literature itself.

The Madness Within Us

1

Schizophrenia as a Philosopher's Concern

During a visit to my office, a young man hesitantly reveals his belief that snakes are living behind the mirror in his college dormitory room and that they are forcing their thoughts into his head. His terror was hidden in the privacy of his own mind for a year, until his failure in his classes led to a confession to his mother and a referral to me. His belief about the snakes is a delusion, a symptom of schizophrenia, and it leads me to prescribe a medication and a course of psychotherapy—and to suggest to him and his parents that he is not ready to return to college. I also tell his parents that this young man, Paul, is at significant risk for suicide and that his cigarette smoking and marijuana use, which they find especially offensive because of their religious beliefs, are part of his illness.

His delusion has many features that mirror other aspects of human thought—creativity, doubt, obsession, conviction, and remembrance. The delusion of snakes living behind the mirror and influencing his thoughts is as creative and dramatic as Harry Potter's struggle with the serpent living behind the walls of Hogwart's Academy. The snakes are constantly writhing and hissing, threatening to come out from the mirror and kill him. The more he stares into the mirror and sees himself, the more convinced he becomes that the snakes are hidden behind the reflection of his face. They hiss that he is a sinner and a failure, and they order him not to leave his room. As a result, he has stopped attending classes and has dropped almost all interactions with his classmates. He leaves his room only to get food and cigarettes.

The snakes are terrifying to Paul, but he also recognizes that he has doubts about them and he understands that the snakes are somehow apart from his normal apprehension of reality. Nonetheless, the extent to which his obsession with the belief seizes his thoughts is remarkable, and he is left unable to concentrate on his classes, with the result that his grades have dropped into the failing range. His conviction about the snakes resists all attempts by his parents and himself to eradicate this belief by appeal to reason. A roommate sees him agitated and offers him a cigarette to try to calm him. He finds that cigarettes help temporarily by restoring his sense of reality and diminishing the intrusion of the snakes into his thinking, and therefore he has begun to smoke regularly. Because his dormitory forbids smoking, he hides in halls and corridors to smoke, where another student, also hiding his smoking, offers him marijuana. The marijuana decreases his anxiety, but when he returns to his room the snakes hiss that the police will imprison him for his illegal drug use. Nonetheless, he starts to use it several times per week.

The medication that I prescribe takes effect quickly, but only partially so. The intensity of his belief about the snakes declines markedly, but it always remains under the surface as a remembrance that can be reactivated and even elaborated, especially during times of stress. Paul is a reserved, often silent young man. He is interested in machinery, which led to his admission to an engineering school. He is happiest cleaning and repairing small motors, and a local lawnmower shop is glad to have him back working part time. His skill level is high enough for him to become an automobile mechanic or even an airplane mechanic, but the pressure of fixing cars or planes quickly and being responsible for their safety is too overwhelming. He is content to fix lawnmowers and generators that can be left in his care for several days. Because good mechanics who will work for low pay are rare, the manager of the local shop is accommodating to his need for work part time, often after the shop is closed and the customers have left.

His parents are distressed that he has little interest in returning to school, which he sees as overwhelming. A couple of attempts at community college are aborted, because he refuses to go to class after his mother has enrolled him. This refusal, sometimes called negativism, is, like the snakes, not amenable to reason. He and I talk within a very restricted framework. He does not generally wish to talk about the snakes, although he was relieved that I understood about them, and he has little to say about the motor repair. He generally uses his time with me to communicate through me to his mother, to let her know that her expectations of him are too demanding, something that he cannot bear to tell her himself. She, in turn, uses her contact with me to grieve for her son whose promise of living as an independent, successful young professional has been dashed. After bringing Paul to me initially, his father has remained silent about his own feelings.

* * * * * *

Schizophrenia, in one form or another, has been recognized as a disturbance in thought and behavior throughout history. An early description of psychosis is in the first Book of Samuel in the Old Testament, where over the course of his several years' reign Saul develops increasingly troubled behavior, ascribed to his failure to obey God's directions through the prophet Samuel's religious injunctions. "Now the spirit of the Lord had departed from Saul, and an evil spirit from the Lord began to terrify him" (I Samuel 16:14). David was initially called to treat the illness because of his skill at playing the lyre: "Whenever the [evil] spirit would come upon Saul, David would take the lyre and play it; Saul would find relief and feel better, and the evil spirit would leave him" (16:23). However, after David's slaying of Goliath, Saul became jealous of him: "From that day on Saul kept a jealous eye on David. The next day an evil spirit of God gripped Saul and he began to rave in his house, while David was playing [the lyre] as he did daily. Saul had a spear in his hand, and Saul threw the spear, thinking to pin David to the wall" (18:9-10).[1]

From the biblical time of Saul, about 1000 BC, until the late nineteenth century, schizophrenia was regarded as a combination of divine inspiration and divine curse. Many of the hermit saints, who lived alone and were deeply suspicious of others, had apocalyptic visions not so dissimilar from our student Paul's snakes. Others who claimed to hear God's voice were burned as heretics. Perhaps the best known is Joan of Arc, whose own description of her voices was transcribed during her trial in 1431 for heresy

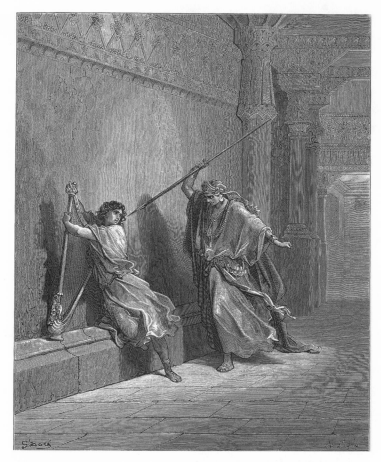

Figure 1-1. *Saul seeks to pin his rival (and therapist) David to the wall.*
Engraving by Gustave Doré (1832–1883).

at the Cathedral in Rouen: "She declared that at the age of thirteen she had
heard a voice from God to help her and guide her. And the first time she
was much afraid.... When she came to France she often heard the
voice.... It seemed to her a worthy voice, and she believed it was sent
from God... 'This voice comes from God, I believe I do not tell
you everything about it, and I am more afraid of failing the voices by
saying what is displeasing to them, than of answering you' " (pp. 42–43).[2]
The trial, which initially concluded with her recantation and her agree-
ment to wear women's clothes instead of men's, was followed by a relapse

when she reappeared in men's clothes, leading to her condemnation and execution.

But many others who have heard voices and had delusions were not recognized as saints or heretics, but seen as deeply disturbed. They became consigned to asylums, which were established in the beginning of the fifteenth century as poverty, criminality, mental disability, and mental illness became the object first of charitable and then of governmental action. The Bethlehem Royal Hospital, founded by the Order of the Star of Bethlehem, admitted its first nine mentally ill patients in 1403. By the nineteenth century when it was taken over by the City of London, it had grown to house many thousands of patients. Visitors were admitted for a penny and could bring poles to poke at the patients. The cockney pronunciation of the hospital's name, "bedlam," became the English word for a scene of uproar and confusion. The final panel of William Hogarth's painting *A Rake's Progress* illustrated the collection of people living in the hospital, crowded into large day rooms. In addition to schizophrenia and mood disorders, many patients were hospitalized because of a mental disorder resulting from infection of their brain by syphilis, brought to Europe from America by the early explorers. The Rake was likely a victim of this common cause of mental illness, which he contracted during his high living in earlier panels of the painting.

Institutionalization resulted in the sorting of individuals into various categories, and physicians who cared for these patients began to increase the precision of their description of schizophrenia as an illness and to differentiate it from other conditions. Emil Kraeplin, the greatest of these, separated schizophrenia from bipolar disorder and senile dementias in the late nineteenth century. He called the illness "dementia praecox," which emphasized that the illness began in early adulthood (praecox), rather than in old age, and involved severe loss of mental function (dementia), as opposed to bipolar disorder, from which the patient would have periods of recovery.

As the illness began to appear as a recognizable entity, not only did its description become more refined but also there was increasing interest in its cause. Early psychiatrists, who worked in the large mental hospitals to which most patients were now consigned, became interested in discerning elements of mental dysfunction that might underlie the complex,

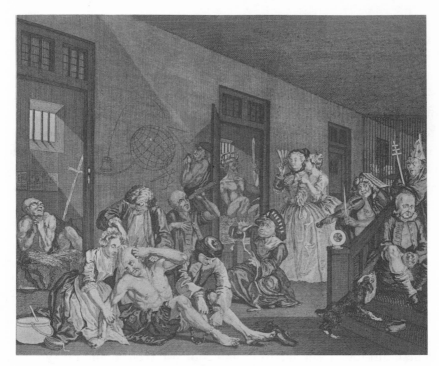

Figure 1-2. *The final panel of eight engravings produced by the English artist William Hogarth in 1735 as A Rake's Progress. The Rake comes to London, jilts his fiancé Sarah Young, and falls into gambling and visiting prostitutes. His descent eventually ends in this scene in the Bethlehem Insane Asylum, where he is comforted by Sarah, surround by grotesquely posturing patients. Several gentile ladies are observing the scene on a social outing.*

bizarre hallucinations, delusions, and behavioral disturbances that the patients exhibited. Unlike most dementias, there were some portions of the mind that appeared intact and others that appeared grossly disturbed. The deterioration in early adulthood, as the bizarre, disorganized thoughts seemed to overwhelm mental functions that had been intact up to that point in life, led Eugen Bleuler in 1908 to name the illness schizophrenia, a splitting apart of the mind. The splitting meant that the mind no longer functioned as a whole, with behavior, emotion, and intellect working together. It did not mean that there were multiple personalities. Bleuler, a contemporary of Kraeplin's, observed that difficulties included autism, affect, association, and ambivalence, sometimes called the four A's.

Autism is the patient's detachment from the world. Paul's isolation in his room and his lifelong inability to make friends are signs of his autism, as well as his belief that only he can hear the snakes. Affect refers to a difficulty regulating emotions such as anger as well as to the emotional withdrawal from others that patients often experience. Paul makes little emotional contact with me, and even his mother saw him as quite distant. He and the owner of the repair shop worked side by side every day, but there seemed to be little camaraderie between them. Once he was over his acute fear of the snakes, he had little to share. Association refers to a disorder in thought, in which irrational symbolic relationships are assumed. For example, Paul thought that an EXIT sign in his dormitory hall might be a communication from the Devil, because of the X contained within it. Ambivalence refers to a patient's inability to commit to a plan of action. Sometimes it is manifest as a stubborn reluctance to follow directions or to conform to other rules of conduct, a trait which leads to their inability to live peacefully in society. Many become street people as a result. Paul's refusal to attend school is an example. Bleuler felt that these traits were the basis of the behavioral disturbance that led to the diagnosis of the illness.

However, it is Bleuler's unnamed fifth A, attention, that seems to be the most elementary of all the dysfunctions. Bleuler noted that persons with schizophrenia have a significant problem in regulating their attention, which he thought was part of their problem in remaining interested and thus part of their affect disturbance. However, he came to realize that it was more complex. Attention is not a unitary property of the brain. To pay attention means to focus interest on some items, while ignoring others that may be louder, brighter, or seemingly more compelling than the object of attention. Reading a newspaper in a crowded restaurant is an example of how attention can be directed to a gray, silent sheet of paper, while around are smells, sights, and sounds that would seem much more interesting.

Patients with schizophrenia in the acute phase of illness are unable to focus their attention, because their interest seems to be grabbed by every stimulus in the environment. As the illness progresses, they seem to defend themselves against this overstimulation by becoming increasingly withdrawn and unresponsive to their surroundings. Without treatment, the withdrawal gradually becomes catatonia, in which they are completely unresponsive and freeze into uncomfortable postures. Bleuler's clinical observations of schizophrenia as a defect in the involuntary aspects of attention are remarkably prescient of a neurobiological understanding of the illness: "Even though uninterested and autistically encapsulated patients pay little attention to the outside world, they register a remarkable number of events of no concern to them. The selection which attention exercises over normal sensory impressions may be reduced to zero, so that almost everything that meets the senses is registered. Thus both the facilitating and inhibitory propensities of attention are disordered."

Catatonic patients, who appear to have withdrawn entirely from the world, had this peculiar hypersensitivity to stimuli in the environment, even as they appeared to be ignoring them: "The patient may reproduce every detail of an event that happened on the ward years before which was of no concern to him, or news items which he heard only in passing, yet at the time he may have appeared preoccupied with himself or staring into a corner, so that it is hard to conceive how he learned about these. One of our catatonics, who for several months was preoccupied with making faces at the wall, after having improved, knew what had happened in the meanwhile in the Boer War."[3]

The concept of the nervous system as the interaction between facilitation and inhibition mediated by the turning on and the turning off of nerve cells would not be fully accepted until 1932, when Sir Charles Sherrington received the Nobel Prize for showing that nerve cells in the brain could inhibit the spinal cord neurons responsible for the knee jerk reflex. Usually, if you tap on your own knee, your leg muscle does not contract, because your brain's concentration on your knee inhibits the reflex. Only when you are distracted, by the doctor's asking you to look away and concentrate on something else, does the reflex appear. As Sherrington put it, "The reflex, therefore, which at first seems a purely excitatory reaction, proves on closer examination to be in fact a commingled excitation and inhibition."[4] Thus, Bleuler's clinical observation of elementary deficits in his patients' behavior was matched by new discoveries of the mechanisms of how the brain works. The possibility of understanding schizophrenia from a neurobiological perspective is part of the reason for the subtitle of this book, "Schizophrenia as a Neuronal Process."

While psychiatrists who specialized in the hospital treatment of psychosis were making observations of the symptoms of patients, neurologists who worked in outpatient clinics were becoming interested in mental illnesses that would come to be called neurosis. The development of humanistic philosophy in Europe led to an increasing appreciation that human behavior was the result of unconscious forces within the mind that were barely controlled by its more conscious elements. As with the visions of earlier saints, the philosophers who created these visions were also isolated, paranoid men. The most striking example is Arthur Schopenhauer, whose paternal grandfather had been in a mental institution and whose father committed suicide. His mother pushed him down the stairs because Goethe called him a genius and she, a writer herself, believed that a family could only have one genius. Schopenhauer lived alone. He was afraid of barbers, who might slit his throat, and kept his smoking pipes in a locked cabinet, to prevent poisoning. Schopenhauer believed that the will, an unconscious force, drove human behavior, and he further believed that his will had been inherited from his father. But, like Bleuler, Schopenhauer was also concerned with how the brain responds to irrelevant stimuli: "I have long held the opinion that the amount of noise which anyone can bear undisturbed stands in inverse proportion to his mental capacity . . . Noise is a torture to all intellectual people . . . . The superabundant display of vitality which takes the form of knocking, hammering, and tumbling things about, has proved a daily torment to me all my life long."[5] He thus seems to be troubled by the same involuntary increase in attentiveness to extraneous stimuli or noise that Bleuler had observed in his patients with schizophrenia.

Sigmund Freud's psychoanalysis was the application of the philosophy of unconscious drives, first described by Schopenhauer, to mental illnesses. Freud suspected that there were problems in the functioning of the brain, which he called constitutional, that interfered with the mind's ability to resolve sexual conflicts in schizophrenia. He therefore recommended against the psychoanalysis of schizophrenia and confined his activities to writing about delusions, based on autobiographical and sometimes fictional accounts. The most famous was an article about the mental illness of Schreber, a German judge who wrote about his persistent delusion that he was being controlled like a puppet. Freud hypothesized that Schreber was afraid of his own homosexual impulses, and that the delusion was the result of his inability to confront and resolve his sexual conflict. Schreber had written in his account of his illness that it had begun with the sudden intrusive thought that he wanted to experience sexual intercourse as a woman.

Just as schizophrenia was in earlier times alternatively ascribed to divine inspiration and divine curse, so too has homosexuality become part of the unsubstantiated myth surrounding schizophrenia. Although Freud's work is frequently referred to as indicating the unconscious roots of schizophrenia in homosexuality, Freud made clear that Schreber did not have schizophrenia and that he did not practice homosexuality. Rather he had paranoia, which Freud differentiated from schizophrenia. Paranoia was an occasional lapse into delusions, whereas schizophrenia was a lifelong inability to move beyond an autistic psychosis. Furthermore, schizophrenia had the additional characteristic of hallucinations, which Freud felt was a more primitive defense mechanism that the paranoid patient's projection of his problems onto others. Freud recognized that individuals could have different elements of paranoia and schizophrenia occurring together, but he did not feel that schizophrenia itself resulted from homosexuality.

Freud concluded:

> Paranoia is precisely a disorder in which a sexual aetiology is by no mean obvious; far from this, the strikingly prominent features in the causation of paranoia, especially among males, are social humiliation and slights. But if we go into the matter only a little more deeply, we shall be able to see the really operative factor in these social injuries lies in the part played by the homosexual components of emotional life. So long as the individual is functioning normally and it is consequently impossible to see into the depths of his mental life, we may doubt whether his emotional relations to his neighbours in society have anything to do with sexuality, either actually or in their genesis. But delusions never fail to uncover these relations and to trace back the social feelings to their roots in a directly sensual erotic wish. So long as he was healthy, Dr. Schreber, too, whose delusions culminated in a wishful fantasy of an unmistakably homosexual nature, had, by all accounts, shown no signs of homosexuality in the ordinary sense of the word.[6]

The psychoanalytic group who pursued the psychological treatment of schizophrenia most avidly was an American group, headed by Harry Stack Sullivan who practiced at Shepperd Pratt Hospital in Maryland. Sullivan was abandoned as a youth and had been taken in by an older man, with whom he had a covert homosexual relationship, because of the criminalization of homosexual conduct. Like Freud, who saw neurotic symptoms as the external manifestation of an internal sexual conflict, Sullivan saw psychotic symptoms as the secondary manifestation of feelings of inadequacy in young people, particularly young men, as they struggled to develop sexual competence and identity. Sullivan believed that "we can isolate by further study a type of situation which I will call the first stage of schizophrenia (because it is so very frequently associated with the second or definite schizophrenia), in which there is a rapid loss of faith in the self and the universe, without the remedial maladjustments or actual remedial processes which go on with most of us when we receive a severe bump in life." Sullivan believed that unfortunate young men, for reasons ranging from intrinsic weaknesses to unfortunate circumstances, including poor parenting, could suddenly and catastrophically lose faith in their ability and in the basic goodness of the world around them. Failure to form stable friendships with their own sex in early adolescence was a developmental sign that the youngster would not be able to accomplish the developmental tasks of later adolescence, when a sense of competence would be required to enter adulthood.

Sullivan had observed such young men transiently lose touch with reality and enter into brief psychotic periods, sometimes during physical illnesses, from which they would seem to recover. He felt that as long as young patients were struggling with the anxiety that there was always the possibility that the personality could be recovered. The most ominous sign was when the struggle stopped as the second stage of schizophrenia emerged: "The second stage of schizophrenia, as it has become formulated in my mind, is somewhat as follows. The individual with serious impairment of the dependability of his self and the universe progresses into a situation in which . . . . a massive transference of blame may occur, as a result of which he progresses into a chronic paranoid state."[7]

The transference of blame is sometimes described as a crystallization, a paranoid solution to the patient's problem, which is malignant, yet stable, with little possibility of recovery. For Paul, the solution to being lonely and frightened, away from home, failing both academically and socially, was that the snakes were influencing his brain. If he gave himself up to them, then they, not he, were responsible for his troubles. Saul's failures as a leader and the alienation of his son Jonathan were easily ascribed to David, the object of his paranoia. Schreber projected his sexual conflicts onto a sun god, whom Freud realized was a projection of his disciplinarian father. Paranoia itself is a common human reaction to overwhelming stress. Conspiracies are the stuff of politics, because in times of national crisis it is easiest to look for external enemies. Sullivan's characterization of the overt symptoms of schizophrenia, particularly paranoia, as natural human developmental processes was the basis of the title of his last book, *Schizophrenia as a Human Process*, compiled by his followers from his speeches and papers after his death. The subtitle to this book thus has a second rationale to acknowledge Sullivan's fundamental insight about how schizophrenia is a pathology that is expressed as part of the normal process of development from adolescence to adulthood.

By the mid-twentieth century, social psychology had characterized schizophrenia, both its sexual conflict and the resultant psychosis, as the product of a sadistic mother and a withdrawn father. The so-called schizophrenogenic mother was the object of a retrospective family therapy, in which the development of psychosis was tied to the pathology demonstrable in the family. Families put enormous stress on their children who have schizophrenia, and vice versa, these children also stress their families. But there has never been evidence that this process is any different from other families with children ill with diabetes, asthma, or mental retardation. Nonetheless, families who brought psychotic children for treatment could expect to be blamed for the illness for which they sought help.

Fortunately, schizophrenia always resists facile characterization. At the peak of the social psychological interpretation, two discoveries intruded into this formulation. First and most obvious was the discovery of antipsychotic drugs. Chlorpromazine, initially synthesized in the nineteenth century as an aniline purple dye extracted from coal tar, was sold to a drug company 70 years later, which discovered that it had some antihistamine properties. It was commonly accepted practice to determine whether new drugs intended for human use were safe, by first administering them to persons with incurable illnesses, like schizophrenia. Therefore, chlorpromazine was administered to patients with schizophrenia in a French mental hospital as part of its early clinical testing as an antihistamine, and found, unexpectedly, to diminish the intensity of their delusions. The first description of the effect once again centered on the patient's involuntary reactions or attention to the environment around them: "He is usually aware of the improvement induced by the treatment but does not show euphoria. The apparent indifference

or the slowing of responses to external stimuli, the diminution of initia-
tive and anxiety without a change in the state of waking and consciousness or of intellectual faculties constitute the psychological syndrome
attributable to the drug."[8] The observation contrasted with the well-
known bedlam that characterized the mental hospitals in which chlorpromazine was first tested, and it also contrasted with the heavy sedation
that the only previously available drugs, the barbiturates, could induce.
Thus, the French psychiatrists, Jean Delay and Pierre Deniker, called
chlorpromazine a neuroleptic agent, their term for the syndrome of
psychomotor slowing, emotional quieting, and affective indifference.
The diminished response to the surrounding environment, now brought
about by a therapeutic drug, is reminiscent of Bleuler's description of his
catatonic patient's solution of standing in a corner and making faces at
the wall. One is a pharmacological situation, the other a self-imposed
isolation, but both attempt to regulate information that the individual
has to register and to respond to.

As remarkable as the discovery of chlorpromazine was for the clinical
treatment of schizophrenia, its interpretation as a neurobiological phenomenon was even more remarkable. The new discipline of neuroscience
was just beginning to reach an understanding of how nerve cells communicate with each other. Synapses, a special connection between nerve
cells, enabled them to communicate through chemicals. These connections between neurons are thus what give the brain its complex interplay
of facilitation and inhibition, a process Bleueler had imagined regulated
attention and Sherrington had already shown could regulate apparently
simple reflexes. Different cells were shown to use different chemicals,
now called neurotransmitters, in their synapses.

Because some aspects of the neuroleptic syndrome resembled
Parkinson disease, in which nerve cells that used dopamine as their
synaptic chemical were lost, Arvid Carlsson proposed and then proved
that chlorpromazine interfered with chemical neurotransmission
mediated by dopamine. The insight that chlorpromazine was blocking
communication between nerve cells at this level led eventually to the
conclusion that drugs, including chlorpromazine, which block the second
of five receptors for the neurotransmitter dopamine (the dopamine D2
receptor), profoundly reduce the intensity of psychotic delusions.
Chlorpromazine and other neuroleptic drugs helped identify the receptor
and, in turn, the receptor was used to identify other drugs that were

effective treatments for psychosis. A complex human phenomenon was seemingly reduced to a simple biological mechanism.

This insight created nearly as much philosophical disturbance for psychiatrists and their patients as the therapeutic effect from these drugs. For psychoanalysts and others invested in the psychotherapy of schizophrenia, the advance was heretical. Chlorpromazine was not

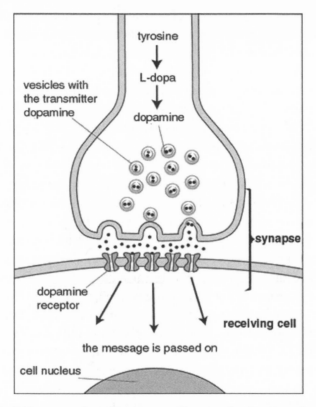

Figure 1-3. *"A message from one nerve cell to another is transmitted with the help of different chemical transmitters. This occurs at specific points of contact, synapses, between the nerve cells. The chemical transmitter dopamine is formed from the precursors tyrosine and L-dopa and is stored in vesicles in the nerve endings. When a nerve impulse causes the vesicles to empty, dopamine receptors in the membrane of the receiving cell are influenced such that the message is carried further into the cell. Arvid Carlsson's research has increased our understanding of the mechanism of several other drugs. He showed that antipsychotic drugs, mostly used against schizophrenia, affect synaptic transmission by blocking dopamine receptors."* Text and diagram from the announcement of Professor Carlsson's Nobel Prize. Karolinska Institute. The Nobel Prize in Physiology or Medicine, 2000.

conceptualized as a dopamine D2 antagonist; rather, psychoanalysts warned that "it separates the ego from the id." In other words, the effectiveness of the drug made the psychological resolution of psychosis impossible, because it diminished the patients' distress that was their motivation for seeking treatment. Sullivan had taught that periods of distress were the only times that patients might resolve their psychosis.

Clinical trials intended to show that psychotherapy without drug treatment leaves patients better in the long term, because they have struggled to understand their psychosis, were resoundingly negative. Most tellingly, recent National Institute of Mental Health investigations of the treatment of schizophrenia have omitted psychotherapy altogether as a treatment modality, under the assumption that most patients will receive some psychological support over the course of the chronic phase of their illness, but that this therapy will not influence the patients' outcome. However, the opposite hypothesis, that early drug treatment of psychosis would be close to curative, because it would prevent people from having the debilitating mental experience of chronic psychosis, has also been regularly negated. The role of dopamine in schizophrenia continues to be debated, but there is little evidence that it is a primary causal factor. Nevertheless, all currently approved treatments block dopamine D2 receptors.

The second discovery that led to a revision of the understanding of schizophrenia had a more ominous origin. Institutionalization and the characterization of schizophrenia as an illness had led some psychiatrists to consider whether the illness was genetically transmitted, because sometimes more than one family member was ill. The question was raised whether sterilization of patients should be performed based on classical epidemiological strategies that isolate and eliminate sources of illness in the population. One of Krapelin's students became the architect of a plan to identify and sterilize people with schizophrenia in Germany. Sterilization of patients in mental institutions indeed continued in a few states in the United States even after the conclusion of World War II and the revelation of the atrocities perpetrated in Europe in the name of eugenics. As repugnant as the eugenics movement now seems, it also fostered a growing interest in investigation of whether human mental illnesses were genetically transmitted.

For schizophrenia, patients' long-term institutionalization led to many births of children conceived by two patients. Most of them were immediately placed for adoption. Tracking their fates led to the discovery that they carried the risk for schizophrenia with them to their adoptive families. Identical or monozygotic twins, who share the same genes, were studied to see if one twin having the illness meant that the other would as well. As the molecular biology of the gene became increasingly understood, it became important to determine whether schizophrenia, which had become the archetypal mysterious mental illness, could be resolved as a genetic illness. Furthermore, if it were genetic, then it was clearly a disease of the biology of the brain, not a dysfunction of the mind wrought by the schizophrenogenic mother.

Paul Meehl, the newly elected president of the American Psychological Association in 1962, stood before his colleagues to deliver his presidential address and challenged devotion to a psychological theory of schizophrenia. He pointed out that no test for schizophrenia based on individual or family psychology was more powerful than the 50% likelihood that schizophrenia in one monozygotic twin would be mirrored by schizophrenia in the other twin.[9]

As the mapping of genes for other illnesses had unprecedented success in revealing their cause, there was great enthusiasm that modern molecular biology would do the same for schizophrenia. But schizophrenia is not inevitably transmitted from parent to child. Its occurrence in two siblings in one family happens often enough (about 1 in 10 cases), however, that these pairs of siblings and their parents can have their chromosomes mapped to see which genetic markers the two ill siblings have in common. Two siblings receiving the same genetic marker from the same parent happens by chance 50% of the time, because each parent has two copies of each genetic marker on two homologous or paired chromosomes; only one of these paired chromosomes is placed into the sperm from the father and the egg from the mother, so that each parent randomly contributes 50% of his or her genes to each sibling. However, if both siblings are ill and the illness comes from a single gene, then the same abnormal variant of the gene should be found in both siblings. In a single family, one cannot tell if the coincidence is due to chance or inheritance. But if many families are studied and if all transmit schizophrenia to their children because of the same genetic variant, then the coincidence exceeds the 50% level. The mathematics developed for examining random events like coin tosses can be used to determine the likelihood that a genetic variant responsible for the illness has been discovered.

Schizophrenia has eluded this insight as well, however. It is not because studies have failed to find genes. To the contrary, over a dozen genes have been found, many of them quite plausibly related to brain dysfunctions involved in schizophrenia. Not a few of them have been found to have significant effects in more than one study. But none has been positive in every study, and none has shown the kind of severe molecular pathology that has been confirmatory of a genetic basis for other illnesses. The problem is not unique to schizophrenia. First, there is a significant non-genetic component. If monozygotic twins who share all their genes have only a 50% chance of both having illness if one has illness, then 50% of the risk must be nongenetic factors like environmental stress, which could influence the baby before or after birth. Second, if a single gene were responsible for illness, then the risk in other siblings (brothers and sisters who are not monozygotic twins who share half their genes) must be 25% or half the risk in monozygotic twins, but the actual risk is only 10%. The fall off in concordance of risk between monozygotic twins and siblings is consistent with there being more than one genetic variant necessary to cause the illness. For common illnesses, like schizophrenia with its prevalence in the population of about 1 in 100 people (because more than one gene is involved and there are environmental factors), the genetic variant of any one of the genes is likely to be found in about 15% of the population. If pathological variants in two genes were necessary for the illness, then almost 30% of the population could be carrying at least one gene for schizophrenia.

Statistical genetics thus changes our notion of schizophrenia in a way that the eugenic psychiatrists could not have imagined. Schizophrenia is now not the result of a rare genetic variant that causes a disaster in the central nervous system and needs to be eradicated by sterilization. Rather, it is the outcome of the combination of common events, including some very common genetic variants in the normal population. Most of the time these genetic variants do not cause illness. Rather, they are part of the diversity in brain function that contributes to differences that make human interactions more complex and rich than the social life of any other species. This genetic insight supports Sullivan's belief that schizophrenia is fundamentally a normal human process.

Genetics is not the only discipline to be frustrated in its attempt to understand schizophrenia. Schizophrenia has been called the graveyard of neuropathologists. Neuropathology, the study of the brain under the microscope after death, was revealing for Alzheimer disease and Parkinson disease, both illnesses that could be traced to the loss of specific types of nerve cells. The findings in schizophrenia have been much less dramatic and less consistent from subject to subject. Similarly, the electroencephalogram (EEG), which is the mainstay of the study of epilepsy, was from its discovery looked upon as the key tool for understanding schizophrenia. A similar hope has been expressed for computerized tomography (CT scans), positron emission tomography (PET scans), and magnetic resonance imaging (MRI). The findings with these techniques mirror the neuropathological findings in their subtleness and limited reproducibility between subjects. These studies are consistent with the insight from genetics that schizophrenia consists of subtle variants in the brain. Thus, Paul has most of his cognitive abilities intact, despite his rather disturbing hallucinations and delusions.

I have chosen to introduce this brief book with the story of the conceptualization of schizophrenia from an evil spirit in biblical times to a genetic variant in modern times, not to disparage these efforts or to bolster the position that the cause can never be found. The amount of knowledge that has been gained is remarkable, as we will see in the next chapters. While the knowledge is incomplete, there is an opportunity to share what has been learned with persons like Paul who are experiencing the illness, their families, and people who care for them. Schizophrenia is unique in that it is the only illness for which people seek help with the complaint that their mind is no longer functioning correctly. Their distress is palpable and their terror, like Paul's about the snakes that are attempting to influence him, is so intense that at first they hide their thoughts. Then, as the illness progresses, they seek help for a symptom that only a human being could articulate. No other animal has the self-observing power to cry out, as Paul did, that its mind has been snatched by an unknown power. Even among the human brain illnesses, it is the most serious illness for which considerable self-observing power remains intact. It is also the illness in which creativity, that seeming unique human capability, becomes part of the pathology as hallucinations and delusions become progressively elaborated over the course of the illness. For those people who have experienced these symptoms or tried to comfort someone who has them, this book is offered as a partial explanation for what may have happened to them. For other readers, there is the possibility that by understanding what has gone awry in schizophrenia, perhaps we can understand better how our brains are constructed and how they function.

Bishop George Berkeley in 1710 pointed out that the brain has no fundamental property of observation. It delivers to our consciousness a stream of information, but we have no independent way of knowing to what extent what is generated comes from the world around us and to what extent our view of the world around us is the product of our own mental function, independent of a surrounding reality. "When we do our utmost to conceive the existence of external bodies [such as people and objects around us], we are all the while only contemplating our own ideas."[10]

Plato made a similar argument about perception over 2,000 years earlier in his parable of the cave in *The Republic*:

> Behold! Human beings living in an underground den, which has a mouth open toward the light and reaching all along the den; here they have been from their childhood, and have their legs and necks chained so that they cannot move, and can only see before them, being prevented by the chains from turning round their heads. They see only their own shadows, or the shadows of one another, which the fire throws on the opposite wall of the cave. And if they were able to converse with one another, would they not suppose that they were naming what was actually before them? To them, the truth would be literally nothing but the shadows of the images.[11]

When I sit in this chair writing to you, what is not clear to either of us is whether each of us is a real person or whether one of us is a figment of the other's imagination. I might be real, but you might be a hallucination that I am having, or vice versa. In more recent times, the mathematician and philosopher Alan Turing proposed that computers could be constructed from a series of fundamental mathematical processes that would produce answers to questions that no human being could discern as not coming from another human being. Philosophers have asked whether such a machine would then be considered human. A human illness in which the ability to discern what is real from what is a functioning by-product of one's own mind might make use of Turing's challenge. The definition of sanity, by analogy with Turing, would be the ability to query one's own perceptions and determine whether they are real or imagined. Most people never bother to ask this question, but many people who have schizophrenia unexpectedly seem to understand intuitively that they have an issue with perceiving reality. For if there is an illness in which reality testing is compromised, Bishop Berkeley might have predicted that an individual with such an illness would have an ontological uncertainty that is more extensive that the average person's. Persons with schizophrenia are certainly more troubled about the issue than other people—Bishop Berkeley excluded. Most of the rest of us are usually oblivious to the issue. Thus, another paradox of schizophrenia is that many of these individuals, like Paul who is terrified by snakes that he knows are not real, have more insight into their ontological predicament than the rest of humanity. It is perhaps therefore also not unexpected that the history of philosophy, and ultimately our understanding of who we are, is very much intertwined with the symptoms of schizophrenia.

2

The Clinical Symptoms of Schizophrenia

Rachel was referred to me after the birth of her third son. She had received a narcotic for pain during the delivery, and after the delivery she seemed odd. Although she could handle the baby just fine, she was emotionally guarded with the nurses to the point that they became worried about her mental status, and she told her obstetrician that she was feeling very anxious in the hospital. She was 28 years old and had not had any previous history of psychiatric difficulty. Her obstetrician called me to say that she thought Rachel "might be getting squirrelly." We agreed that I would see her the next morning.

The Diagnosis of Schizophrenia

We have not yet discussed how the diagnosis of schizophrenia is made. When the treatment was limited to chronic hospitalization in the nineteenth century, the diagnosis was made on the basis of severe behavioral disturbance. Early in the twentieth century as psychotherapists became more interested in schizophrenia, the diagnosis broadened. Sometimes patients receiving psychoanalysis would develop delusions about the therapist that seemed to go beyond even the usual intense transference feelings that all patients have for therapists. Instead of improving, their behavior would begin to deteriorate. They were termed pseudo-neurotic schizophrenics, because they initially appeared to have a neurosis, but actually they had schizophrenia. Some psychiatrists began to diagnosis schizophrenia in any patient who made them feel odd or uncomfortable.

Overlabeling of patients became a civil rights concern in the mid-twentieth century. If patients could be hospitalized for long periods of time because of a diagnosis of schizophrenia, then a psychiatrist would seem to have the ability to act as judge and jury in determining a patient's liberty. A romanticization of schizophrenia as an alternative mental lifestyle partly contributed to the idea that psychiatrists might be acting high handedly to label others as ill, simply because they saw reality in a different way. In fact, in the Soviet Union, some political dissidents were incarcerated in mental hospitals on the basis that anyone who held alternative political beliefs must be insane.

Researchers in the 1970s had already begun to confront the problem of rigorous diagnosis and as genetic and neurobiological research advanced, it was increasingly more important that findings be comparable in groups of patients across the world. It was disquieting that American psychiatrists were diagnosing schizophrenia at twice the rate of their British and European colleagues. With the introduction of lithium carbonate as a specific treatment for bipolar manic-depressive mood disorder, the distinction of this diagnosis from schizophrenia became even more relevant for medical treatment. In this climate, Eli Robbins at Washington University in St. Louis established the Research Diagnostic Criteria to attempt to return the diagnosis of schizophrenia to the rigorous distinctions that had characterized Kraeplin's work at the beginning of the twentieth century.[1] As a young psychiatrist, Dr. Robbins underwent psychoanalysis as part of his training. He developed a psychosis and later transient loss of sight, which were attributed to a deepening neurotic transference to his psychoanalyst. He eventually consulted a neurologist, who diagnosed multiple sclerosis, which sometimes presents initially as psychosis and loss of sight. He resolved that his research and clinical practice would improve psychiatric diagnosis.

The American Psychiatric Association decided to follow suit and replaced its simple list of diagnoses in its *Diagnostic and Statistical Manual*, then in its second edition (DSM-II), with a set of specified criteria for schizophrenia and other illnesses, based on the Research Diagnostic Criteria. DSM-III was then replaced by DSM-III-R (revision) and then by DSM-IV and DSM-IV-TR (text revision), all within 25 years. DSM-V is now in the first stage of preparation, and the distinction between schizophrenia and bipolar mood disorder continues to be a major driving force behind these revisions.

There is no single symptom that defines schizophrenia to the exclusion of all other mental illnesses and therefore the criteria begin by looking at its most unusual characteristic symptoms as a group. Five categories of symptoms are described and the patient must have at least two for a 1-month period. The first is delusions. Delusions are persistent beliefs that are not true. Paul's belief that the snakes are trying to influence his mind is an example, called thought insertion, which is common in schizophrenia. Rachel would soon reveal to me that she believed that aliens in spaceships orbiting in a faraway galaxy were influencing her. Hallucinations, generally auditory hallucinations such as voices, are a second category. These need to be more than a word or two. People in a variety of stressful circumstances sometimes hear their name being called; that does not suffice as a hallucination. In their most extreme form, the voices converse with each other in running, derogatory comments about the patient. Hallucinations in this form are considered sufficient by themselves as a characteristic symptom of schizophrenia. The snakes' comments about Paul's sins are an example of auditory hallucinations. Rachel felt that the nurses were whispering about her, which was plausible, but she also felt that her sister had crept back into the hospital after visiting hours and that she could hear her voice as well. That phenomenon, which she knew could not possibly be true, qualified as an auditory hallucination. The patient only has to hear the voices or have the delusions, not believe that they are real. Many patients have delusions or hallucinations that they know are not true and are instead based in their own thoughts. Bishop Berkeley would be fascinated by the strength of their conviction that the voices are not real.

Disorganized speech and grossly disorganized or catatonic behavior, the third and fourth symptoms of schizophrenia, are not as common as hallucinations and delusions. They are more likely to occur in individuals who have not been treated for many years. Negatives symptoms, the last of the five characteristic symptoms, are commonly observed. The other symptoms are positive, that is, symptoms that do not appear in most

normal persons. Negative symptoms are the absence of a normal behavior. An example is alogia, the absence of thought content in speech.
Rachel always has things to say, but Paul has alogia. Alogia does not
mean silence. Paul will always answer if spoken to, and his speech always
makes sense. What it lacks is anything other than minimal content. He is
unable to summon forth material of interest to himself or anyone else.
Work is okay, things are okay at home, he is okay, but he never expresses
interest in what he is doing, nor does he reflect about what has happened
to him, nor does he show curiosity about his future. He is truly empty, as
far as we can tell from speech. His lack of interest in accomplishing
anything, termed avolition, and his reserved or flattened affect are
other negative symptoms.

Any of the five characteristic symptoms can occur in normal people.
A small percentage of the population hears voices regularly. Paranoid
delusions are the normal stuff of politics, as we said earlier. Negative
symptoms are difficult to distinguish from normal teenage behavior.
These symptoms therefore do not constitute an illness in themselves,
and, in accord with the genetics and neurobiology that we reviewed in
the last chapter, they are better viewed as variants of normal thought
and behavior. Thus, there is a second major criterion for schizophrenia, which is social and occupational dysfunction. For Paul, who
was hoping to be an engineer, returning to his part-time high school
job repairing motors was clearly below his expected level of functioning, had he not become ill. For Rachel, the diagnosis was more
difficult. She had a master's degree in literature and had expected to
teach or write after she had her children. We assessed her carefully to
determine competence to care for her children, but we relied on her
own mother for some supervisory help, made sure that the three boys
were seen frequently, and that they could access their grandmother
directly.

Psychoses can occur briefly for a number of reasons, but schizophrenia
has always been conceptualized as a lifelong illness. Both for Paul, who
was smoking marijuana which can be laced with any number of halluci-
nogens, and for Rachel, whose illness began after receiving narcotics, we
hoped that the psychoses were drug induced and that they would disappear as the drug left their brains. Even within the families of persons
with schizophrenia, some family members will have brief psychoses
during the stress of transitions like entering school, and we want to

avoid giving such a person a label generally reserved for a chronic mental illness. Therefore, the third criterion is signs of the illness for at least 6 months. Unfortunately, both Paul and Rachel eventually fulfilled that criterion. As we got to know them better, we understood that the illness had begun much earlier, but that history was difficult to elicit in first interviews.

The final three criteria are used to distinguish schizophrenia from other mental illnesses. The first distinction is between schizophrenia and mood disorders. During the peaks of mania and the valleys of depression, individuals with these disorders can become psychotic as well. Diagnosticians must evaluate which of the two illnesses predominates and, specifically, whether psychotic symptoms can be seen in the absence of mood symptoms. Rachel was depressed in the postpartum period and her family was asked by friends if she might be bipolar, because some patients with bipolar disorder, although not usually those with prominent psychosis, do much better than most patients with schizophrenia. But, in fact, she had periods of psychosis that occurred when there was no depression. If the depression or mania and the psychosis almost always occur together, then a diagnosis of schizoaffective disorder is made, essentially an illness that has the features of both schizophrenia and bipolar disorder. I prefer to make a distinction between schizophrenia and bipolar disorder if at all possible, because it helps guide the treatment. The second distinction is between drug-induced psychoses and schizophrenia. Paul stopped using marijuana when he returned home, because he lost his source of the drug, and Rachel had received narcotics only during delivery. Therefore, drugs were not an issue for our two patients. The third distinction is psychosis during a childhood developmental disorder. We will discuss psychosis in children in a subsequent chapter.

Our final diagnostic task was to subtype Rachel and Paul. Subtyping helps determine what psychological approach to take with the patient. Paul's deep suspicion of the snakes and Rachel's suspicion of the nurses led to a paranoid subtype for each. Paranoid schizophrenia, as opposed to catatonic, disorganized, undifferentiated, or residual, is the most common type. Paranoid patients are generally the brightest, because, rather than simply deteriorating, they had the mental ability to go through the stage of reorganizing themselves to shift the blame to others, as Sullivan described.

Finding the Neurobiology of Schizophrenia

None of these signs and symptoms immediately calls to mind any sort of simple neuronal process. Many fields of medicine have taken advantage of animal models to reach biological explanations of human illnesses, such as diabetes whose pathology was elucidated in dogs whose pancreases were removed. Because of schizophrenia's unique pathology in the process of thought itself, there is no obvious animal model, or at least we have no sure means of detecting whether animals have disordered thoughts. Medicine has also relied on removing the offending organ and examining it under the microscope, an indispensable tool for determining that pneumonia was caused by a bacterial infection of the lung. However, it is wisely considered unethical to remove brain tissue during life, when an active disease process might be discoverable. Examination of the brain postmortem has not revealed an abnormality that obviously causes the full symptomatic picture of schizophrenia. Thus, the traditional tools of medicine have not been entirely helpful for elucidating the cause of schizophrenia. Neither have some of the newer tools such as genetic investigation or some of the newer techniques of medical imaging, as we mentioned in Chapter 1.

What schizophrenia does have in common with other medical fields is that understanding the brain abnormalities that result in schizophrenia has value for explaining not only schizophrenia itself but also for giving us some insight into how the brain normally works to process information into thought. Illnesses are natural experiments in which a malfunction often serves to identify a normal function that cannot otherwise be discerned. Our brain function is normally unrecognizable to us, because as Bishop Berkeley pointed out, it is the tool of our perception. But the person with schizophrenia, who recognizes himself that his brain is malfunctioning, is an example of how the brain can malfunction just enough so that the person can articulate that there is a problem, and we can use their insights to learn something about how our own brains work.

There are two aspects of the abnormalities associated with schizophrenia that we shall be considering in the next chapters. The first question to answer is how the brain's processing of information goes astray. The answer to that question will identify neurons that are malfunctioning in schizophrenia. The second question is to determine why these neurons are malfunctioning. You might recognize that if we had a definitive answer to either one of the questions then we would have a solid piece of evidence for use in answering the other. If in answering the first question, we came to understand that schizophrenia as a whole or one of its symptoms was caused by the failure of a particular nerve cell function, then we would look for genetic abnormalities associated with that function or viruses that attack the nerve cells involved, or the like. On the other hand, if we knew that a specific gene or virus causes schizophrenia, then we would examine all the nerve cell functions affected by that gene or virus to determine which of these functions was the critical one for producing symptoms of schizophrenia. Even if we believe that stress caused schizophrenia, we would still want to know which nerve cell functions fail under stress and which of the stress hormones causes that failure.

As we know from Chapter 1, schizophrenia does not have simple answers and we do not have a definitive psychological explanation that leads from hallucinations and delusions to the failure of a specific nerve cell and a specific function of that nerve cell. Nor do we have a definitive pathogen—gene, virus, stress, or something else—that we can use to identify which elements fail. There was hope that the early apparent success of chlorpromazine and related drugs would identify a specific dysfunction. While the mechanism of the drug effect was successfully elucidated as the dopamine D2 receptor, malfunction of that receptor has not been confirmed as the cause of schizophrenia.

In this chapter we will concentrate on one element of the psychological pathology of schizophrenia, an abnormality in sensory processing that has been noted in schizophrenia, and we will attempt to identify the psychological and neurobiological aspects of its pathology in schizophrenia. Wherever possible in this chapter and the next, we will use psychological and biological information together to try to converge on an identification of the abnormality. Because neither source of information is certain, there is the possibility that their convergence will not produce a description of the neuronal abnormalities that is any more accurate than either of the uncertain sources. This method has led to many tales of the cause of schizophrenia, likely too many for all of them to be correct. With this caution in mind, we will try to construct as good a theory as we can and then, like all scientific theories, subject it to as rigorous a test as possible.

The brain has long seemed intuitively to be hierarchical. It seems to do simple things, like responding to unexpected sounds, and complicated things, like deciding if our mother was really right about our being ungrateful children. Furthermore, we know that many animals can do simpler things as well or even better than we do, but we suspect that more complicated tasks, like reading, are beyond their mental abilities. However, a glance at a rat's brain and our brain shows that our brain is not radically different. Rather, it seems as if our brain has simply developed as a larger and more elaborated rat brain, with the rat brain having all the basic elements. Thus, it would seem reasonable to assume that the human brain somehow derives its complex functions from simple ones.

Therefore, if we seek to understand how the brain malfunctions in schizophrenia, then we could begin not by trying to describe in exquisite detail all the ways in which persons with the illness fail to think correctly, but rather by trying to find a very simple thing that they cannot do. Responses to simple sensory stimuli have long been of interest to investigators of schizophrenia, as we mentioned in the previous chapter. More complicated thoughts, such as how you think about your mother, begin and end in the brain itself, and therefore as an outside observer I have no way to determine when you started your thought or how long it lasted. After all, I cannot be sure about the veracity of my own thoughts and therefore how can I be sure about yours? However, if we both listen to a simple sound or look at a simple object, I can be reasonably sure that both of us have started from the same point, just as if we were chained next to each other in Plato's shadowy cave.

Elementary Brain Dysfunction in Schizophrenia

The earliest observers of how people with schizophrenia seemed to react to their environment noted a peculiarity in the ability of persons with schizophrenia to appear unaware of the environment and yet overly responsive to it. Eugen Bleuler first developed the concept of an attentional dysfunction in schizophrenia in his essay on attention in schizophrenia, which was quoted in the previous chapter.

Rachel not only hears voices but she hears noises as well, noises that her family members also hear but have learned to ignore. She hears screaming all the time, and she sometimes wanders the neighborhood to find out who is screaming. When my colleague Merilyne Waldo suggested to her that it might be the traffic, she told us that her mother had said the same thing. There is a busy corner near the front of her house, and there are always cars stopping and then accelerating away. My wife and I experienced the very same perceptual abnormality ourselves on the night we brought our first son home from the hospital. We put the baby to bed and tried to sleep ourselves, but I heard screaming. I checked on the baby, and he was asleep. Then my wife heard it too. We checked again. Then we listened at the door. The screaming must be coming from another apartment, and we wondered if we should call the police to alert them to child abuse, but we knew that no other couples with babies lived in the building. Finally, when the traffic on the highway in front of the building stopped at 2 a.m., we understood how two very anxious, hyper-vigilant new parents can misinterpret the world around them.

For Rachel, the problem is not a single stressful night. It is a lifelong problem, which she has struggled with since she was a teenager, long before the onset of her illness at 28. She could never concentrate at school. The least noise grabbed her attention. As she put it, "My mind has to be here, it has to be there, I can't concentrate on anything." Unlike a typical child with attention-deficit disorder (ADD), whose attention is rarely captured, her attention was captured by everything, from the traffic squeaking to the refrigerator cycling on and off, to the neighbor's ongoing argument next door. As a result, she could concentrate on very little.

Paul, on the other hand, seems to be aloof from his environment. When he was first ill and worried about the snakes, I wondered if their voices arose out of noises around him in the dormitory. He acknowledged that the noise of the dormitory was exquisitely painful, but he could not connect it to the snakes. Now he seems withdrawn. When I walk out to get him in the waiting room, he seems oblivious to the people around him. He has constructed a psychological shell around himself, a solution many patients use to shield themselves from their otherwise over-whelming environment.

The most dramatic experience of the phenomenon of seeming to ignore the environment is catatonia, a rarely seen syndrome in schizophrenia today. The patient gradually stops responding to environmental stimuli and then eventually stops moving altogether. In the most advanced cases, the person suddenly freezes. If he is moved passively, then he may retain the position into which he is moved, a symptom termed "waxy flex-ibility." These patients can often be drawn back to awareness by family members and sometimes even a familiar physician, which leads to the supposition that they may be faking their symptoms. They are not, and it is sometimes shameful to watch medical personnel positioning them in uncomfortable poses or raising their arms over their faces to see if they will prevent their arms from hitting their eyes, a misguided attempt to uncover what they believe to be malingering.

Patients with catatonia have hyperactive electroencephalographic activity, consistent with the minds being quite active, rather than asleep or anesthetized. They respond to barbiturates and benzodiazepines, drugs that are sedatives, with a paradoxical "awakening," in which they resume normal movement. This paradoxical response suggests that they have actively withdrawn from the world around them, perhaps to inhibit their response to stimuli. When the barbiturate or benzodiazepine partially inhibits their brain's responsiveness, they lose this withdrawal and tem-porarily resume normal interaction. They often report that they were fully aware, indeed acutely hyper-aware, of their surroundings during the cat-atonia. Catatonia takes several years to develop and most persons receive drug treatment before it becomes an obvious symptom. I have occasionally seen it develop in patients from religious families who resist treatment and expend great effort to interact with their loved one, who is descending into deepening catatonia. The otherworldly trance adds to the spiritual mys-tique of their loved one's experience.

Schizophrenia as a Sensory Disturbance

The modern explanation of sensory disturbance in schizophrenia has an equally apocalyptic origin, however. During World War II, with radar in its infancy, the British relied on visual spotters to detect and identify airplane movement across the English Channel coming from Europe. Returning British planes needed airfields cleared and prepared to receive them. Invading Nazi planes required a quite different response—the airfields needed to bring all available planes to the runways to take off to fight the incoming bombers. Britain called on experimental psycholo-gists to help improve the ability of plane spotters to identify the aircraft quickly and at great distance, when features might be difficult to discern.

Donald Broadbent, Britain's great experimental psychologist, quickly learned that there were two separate aspects to the task.[2] The first was a detection problem: to be able to see the plane when it was just a dot in the clouds. The second was a classification problem: to be able to check identifying features such as aircraft shape and insignia to determine what kind of aircraft the dot represented. People concentrating on detection were poor at classification and, vice versa, those who concentrated on classification were poor at detecting aircraft early. Broadbent divined that these were two separate features of perception and that people should be trained to do each independently. Detectors needed to be hypervigilant to the least hint of a plane and, while performing that task, they would not do well at classifying the planes, whereas those classifying planes had to be less hypervigilant and instead more concerned with careful checking of features.

Broadbent saw the two different types of tasks as distinct steps in the earliest stages of perception. He reasoned that the part of the brain that makes decisions, such as which plane is which, has limited capacity and that the brain needed mechanisms to prevent itself from being overwhelmed with stimuli. If the brain were always trying to process every stimulus fully, its decision-making capacity would be quickly overwhelmed and greatly slowed. One problem is how to decide prior to full processing which stimulus is important enough to be processed. Broadbent realized that the primary filter needed to have a very simple principle. It did not need to eliminate all extraneous stimuli, but it needed to eliminate a substantial fraction of them, with little processing requirement. He proposed that if stimuli could be processed briefly to determine if they were being repeated, then the filter could simply eliminate those that were repetitive. Repeated information has little significance and hence the brain can ignore it. Repeated information generally has little significance. Only advertisers, politicians, and educators seem to have missed this basic lesson in human neurobiology.

Broadbent's concepts influenced psychiatrists to think once again about sensory perception in schizophrenia. The dominant thinking in the field was psychoanalytic, which held that schizophrenia was the failed attempt to deal with sexual impulses. What if the problem were much simpler? The struggle might be against a flood of unwanted sensory stimuli. The clinical observation of acutely ill patients suggested that they indeed could be overwhelmed by stimuli in their environment.

Rachel's problems in the hospital became obvious to her within a week of her discharge. Rachel is a very bright woman who was very close with her sister. Rachel was brighter, but her sister was more outgoing. They protected each other in high school, Rachel helping her younger sister with her homework and Susan making sure that Rachel always felt included in their social circle. Rachel went away to school with a scholarship, whereas Susan attended a nearby college. At college, Rachel's symptoms first became manifest as anxiety. She controlled it with cigarettes, alcohol, and marijuana. Because of her intelligence, she was able to continue her progress in school, unlike Paul whose psychosis was more intense and interfered with his more average intellectual abilities. Rachel's attractiveness was also helpful in her career and she was seduced by several teaching assistants, who would also give her the liquor she needed.

She knew that she could not continue at the Ivy League college at her present rate of consumption of drugs and she therefore returned home to get her master's degree at the same university that her sister attended. An introduction to a roommate of her sister's boyfriend led to marriage. She felt better during her pregnancies, which is not uncommon among women who are developing schizophrenia, and the postpartum blues were seen as normal by her family and her obstetrician. The delusional experience she had was not new to her, but her reaction surprised her. She had always been hypersensitive to noise. At school, she found the libraries calming. She hated the noise in the dormitories and was a strong advocate of enforcement of rules about parties, record players, and musical instruments. Occasionally in the library she heard voices that she initially thought were whispering, and she whimsically decided she was the next Joan d'Arc. She fell in with some New Age spiritualists who assumed she had experienced the voices on LSD, which indeed produces hallucinatory experiences.

In the hospital, however, something was different. The noise seemed overwhelming and she could not control her response to it. Many things had changed. Her sister was upset with her for having a third child and she felt criticized and angry at her sister. She could hear her sister's critical remarks ringing through her ears. The hospital was undergoing remodeling, and it was indeed noisy. As an older mother, her delivery had been more complicated, and she had required anticholinergic drugs and narcotics that also had psychotomimetic properties.

We talked several times about what had happened and why. What had happened had been more ominous than her earlier experiences with hypersensitivity to noise. This time she had the distinct impression that the nurses were talking about her, and her sister's voice was prominent among them. However, the voice was much more critical and derogatory than her sister's had ever been, and it commented on all of her imperfections. Her only response was to withdraw from all contact with the nurses, leading to their correct appraisal that something odd was happening to her. As she became more comfortable with me, she was able to reconstruct exactly what had happened to her. However, reconciliation with her sister was more difficult. Just as Sullivan described, she reconstituted the failed parts of her personality by shifting the blame to her sister, whom she now viewed as domineering and selfish.

Peter Venables realized that Broadbent's model for detecting airplanes could be applied to understanding the onset of schizophrenia.[3] There are two aspects to sensory dysfunction in schizophrenia, reflective of the two mechanisms involved in the model. First, there is the sensation of being overwhelmed, with heightened sensitivity to the environment. Patients were being flooded by stimuli because of the absence of a fully functional filtering mechanism. Venables termed their condition "input dysfunction." More commonly, we use the term "sensory gating deficit." The control or gating of stimuli reaching the brain's processing centers is lost, as Bleuler had earlier proposed. Patients might then withdraw, either voluntarily by being isolative or involuntarily through catatonia, to escape this flood of information. The second part of Broadbent's model is equally important. If the second step that makes decisions is overwhelmed, then we would expect to see miscategorization of stimuli. Simply being overwhelmed might be terrifying or might be a pleasant psychedelic experience, but miscategorization would be problematic for behavior. This element was also present for Rachel. Her sister had come to the nursing station and in fact Rachel could overhear her talking with the nurses, but she could not be sure exactly what she said to them or what they said to her. But she seemed to hear the word "crazy." She resented being called crazy, although she admitted that she did not know that her sister had actually said that. Her sister claimed that she probably said something much more benign, such as: "Things look crazy here today with all this remodeling." It was remarkable that this single misperceived interchange, in the midst of the stress of the postpartum period and the hospital environment, was sufficient to alter the course of Rachel's life and her relationship with her sister.

Sometimes, for simple matters, we can help patients therapeutically by intervening in the perceptual process. Rachel once called me from her cell phone during her scheduled appointment. "I can't come to the office, because I look too insane," she said. She had been to every biweekly appointment for a year and had done well. If she could not come when she was sick, her capability to care for her children might be in jeopardy. I told her to come to the quadrangle outside my office in 10 minutes. I decided to help her see how she looked from the point of a view of a perceptual problem. "You don't look as bad as you think," I said when I saw her. "Your shirt is not tucked in, your hair is not combed well, and you don't have your lipstick on. Can you handle those three things?" She walked to a corner, arranged herself with a pocket mirror, and said that she was ready to come upstairs.

Patients often suspect when they have misperceived something. Rachel hears voices when she vacuums her house. Although she does not say that she can pinpoint the noise from the vacuum cleaner as the cause of the misperception, she has learned that the voices that she hears while vacuuming may not be real. Nevertheless, she cannot be certain and therefore she calls her mother, whose voice she hears, to make sure that she is not in her house, but in her own house instead. Someone who treats people for schizophrenia must be prepared for similar phone calls, as suspicions and uncertainties come and go, during the course of the treatment. When a patient calls me at an inopportune time, I recall that Bishop Berkeley was not always sure about reality.

For more complicated misperceptions, those that lead to longer-term delusions and hallucinations, it can be more difficult to alter the misperception. Many people who first learn to treat people with schizophrenia are told not to bother to try to understand the psychological meaning of the person's hallucinations and delusions, because such understanding is difficult to achieve and, even when achieved, rarely leads to their alleviation. They are taught instead to concentrate on helping patients with meaningful activities in their daily life, like their ability to hold a job. Some instruction on the nature of the hallucinatory experience is helpful for patients, because their ability to hold a job may depend upon their avoiding misperception of the work situation and their coworkers. Paul and I began working on his interaction with customers, because the shop's owner wanted him to care for the shop so that he could take a vacation. We worked on interpreting customers' frustrations with delays while he waits for parts to arrive as not being personal attacks on him.

Strategies to improve filtering by psychotherapeutic or psychopharmacological intervention are discussed in Chapters 5 and 6, but practical advice can be very helpful. For example, Paul was quite welcome to stay at his parents' home, but on Saturday evening they liked to have cocktail parties. Since it was known in the neighborhood that he lived at home, it was important to his parents that he come down from his room to greet their friends. Cocktail parties are classic settings for misperception, even above the effects of the liquor. Multiple conversations occur and the person with schizophrenia feels overwhelmed by the amount of sensory information. Just like Rachel, Paul complains: "I hear all the people talking at once. I have trouble understanding anyone." I taught Paul to approach the problem of the cocktail party as an information-processing problem. He learned to take the back stairway from his bedroom to the kitchen rather than coming directly into the living room, and then to gradually work his way around the edges of the party. When he had greeted everyone, then he knew that he had done his job for his parents.

Linus Pauling, the only person to receive two Nobel Prizes, one for Chemistry and one for Peace, became convinced that niacin deficiency was the cause of schizophrenia and that megavitamin treatment would reverse the illness. Patients reportedly improved in a therapeutic community based on niacin therapy, although rigorous tests in more traditional medical settings were negative. The description of the group setting in the therapeutic community is quite informative, however. Patients were initially given only one task: to be able to name all the members of the community. Every morning, a group circle was formed to assist patients in learning everyone's name. This simple technique, cleverly devised by Pauling's collaborator, is a good one to help patients feel calmer and more connected to the people around them.[4]

Input dysfunction can so overwhelm mental function that it is tempting to conceptualize all of schizophrenia as the result of chronic input dysfunction. However, it may be that the elementary dysfunction is not the root cause at all. By analogy, we do not think that someone fails a test because he cannot not see the boxes in which the marks are to be placed. Similarly, these elementary perceptual dysfunctions could be the result of defects in the higher-level functions that should normally engage these perceptual mechanisms. A psychologist once hypnotized subjects to believe that they could not hear and then placed them in a social gathering.[5] Many of them became suspicious about what others around them were saying about them. The example illustrates that human perception is complicated and can be controlled "top down." In this example, elementary perception works fine, but its engagement is altered by the hypnotic suggestion.

Perhaps the underlying problem in schizophrenia is not perceptual, but rather is motivational. We normally engage filters because we care deeply about the world around us and we want to perceive some element of it correctly, one that we are trying to concentrate on. However, a person with schizophrenia, perhaps because of their interest in their inner thoughts, perhaps because of their disinterest in life generally, may not desire to pay attention to the outside world and therefore may not engage all the neuronal circuitry appropriate for perception. Clinical lore includes the tale of a night when one of the buildings of a mental hospital burned down. Yet even the sickest patients quickly mobilized to fight the fire effectively, their symptoms held in abeyance. When the fire was finally put out, the superintendent invited the patients to the dining hall for hot chocolate but before the evening was over, many of them had resumed all their bizarre behaviors. The issue of top-down control of attention versus bottom-up is not resolvable, because the brain works both ways.

Another way to frame the issue is by the analogy to a computer diagnostic. When a computer cannot remember words, we do not try to test it with a dictionary. Instead, we give it the simplest signals we can, electrical pulses, to determine which memory chip has malfunctioned. If we wish to view schizophrenia as a neurobiological illness, then we must move as close as we can to a neuronal level or computer chip level of analysis. However, if we can use a simple function to discover a neuronal dysfunction, it does not mean that the neuronal dysfunction's impact is limited to simple sensory processing. It may be that the same type of neuron is malfunctioning in other brain areas during more complicated tasks. The value of the sensory gating dysfunction hypothesis is that it is particularly amenable to neurobiological analysis. The input can be repeated sensory stimuli, the very situation that Broadbent's filter was conceived to act upon. An advantage of these simple sensory paradigms is that they do not rely directly on the subject's interest or motivation. As long as the subject is reasonably awake and cooperative, meaningful data can be obtained.[6]

The symptoms of schizophrenia, including hallucinations and delusions, are symptoms of psychological dysfunction. It is our goal in the characterization of schizophrenia as a neuronal illness to determine if there is a corresponding brain or neuronal dysfunction. Input dysfunction and sensory gating dysfunction are hypothetical bridging terms. They presuppose a mechanism that works in the brain to change the response to sensory stimuli that will also result in a perceptual change in the mind. There are surprisingly few such correlations. Philosophically, some people doubt that there is any way of proving such correspondence. The French philosopher Descartes, who postulated that only faith could connect the biology of the body with the soul's belief in God, is often held responsible for the origin of the mind–brain dichotomy. Some feel that the shift in terms between psychological and neuronal dysfunction prevents rigorous proof that one depends on the other. Others feel that we are simply trying to impose our simplistic hypotheses on a system that is too complex to be resolved. The brain's 10 billion neurons operate in systems that we do not yet understand. Indeed, say some, if the brain were simple enough to understand, it would not be a very good brain.

Schizophrenia is not a condition that has been seriously examined philosophically, despite our contention that philosophers have been afflicted with it. It has properties that any philosophy of the mind must consider. First, there is self-observation of the loss of mental powers, the problem in sensory perception, and the resistance of many delusions to reason. Second, the illness's genetic transmission holds the promise that discrete biological elements responsible for each of these dysfunctions can be identified. This latter point is the one that we will examine more fully, because results of investigations from mental dysfunction to analogous neuronal dysfunction to underlying genetic variance form one piece of evidence for the soundness of the correspondence of psychology and neurobiology. But as exhilarating as the descent to the genetic level may be, it does not follow that we can then easily trace the way back and demonstrate rigorously that what we have learned genetically is responsible in a comprehensible, mechanistic way for the mental dysfunction. Indeed, we will later have to confront some evidence that this is not the case.

Excitation and inhibition are neuronal mechanisms that have specific biological properties that we will need to demonstrate, not just postulate. That is problematic for human neurobiologists because many of the tools of neurobiology are destructive of brain tissue. Opening the skull, removal of living brain tissue for study, and injection of drugs and toxins and radioactive tracers, are all common techniques for neurobiologists. Obviously, these techniques are not possible for human studies. It would not be a problem if there were a well-accepted animal model of schizophrenia, but the perception of reality is a uniquely human concern. Therefore, we need to somehow improvise a related series of animal and human investigations that reveal to us the neurobiology of sensory gating and then help us identify the specific deficit in human beings. We take up that task in the next chapter.

3

The Neurobiology of Sensory Gating Deficits

The concept of sensory gating that we introduced in the last chapter is well suited to bridge basic neurobiology and the human mental dysfunction that results in schizophrenia. This chapter assumes that you have no background in how the nervous system is organized or how it functions, but that you are curious about how schizophrenia might arise from the dysfunction of nerve cells. Brain biology is not simple, and therefore a somewhat lengthy description follows with the goal of allowing you to learn enough about nerve cells and their circuits to then understand how psychosis might arise from their dysfunction.

Nerve Cells and Their Connections

Nerve cells are the largest cells in the body. They have a cell body with tremendous capacity to produce energy from the sugar glucose and with similar capacity to synthesize protein for their growth and repair. They receive and transmit information and otherwise have no function. They cannot divide into new cells, and therefore they form permanent stores of information, although the form of that storage is unknown. What is known is the common mechanisms by which they receive, process, and transmit information.[1] Nerve cells have large stores of potassium ion inside their cell membrane and they are bathed in a solution of sodium ions, similar to the sea. When they open pores in their membrane and sodium flows in and potassium flows out, an electrical impulse is generated. The timing of the pores opening and closing means that the impulse, about a tenth of a volt, lasts less than a thousandth of a second. The pulse of electricity, called an action potential, travels all over the cell, but particularly down its longest fiber, called its axon. At the end of the axon is a bulb called a presynaptic terminal. It contains packets of chemicals, generally a specific neurochemical of a class called neurotransmitters, based on the function we are about to observe. When the action potential reaches the presynaptic terminal, it releases several packets of the neurotransmitter. The presynaptic terminal is closely bound to a postsynaptic density, which is a protein structure on another nerve cell. These proteins receive the neurotransmitter and then activate several cell processes, including opening the first of the pores that will cause electrical currents to flow across the membrane of their nerve cell. We say that there is chemical neurotransmission from the presynaptic terminal of one nerve cell to the postsynaptic density of the other cell. Most of the postsynaptic densities are on a second kind of fiber that comes from the nerve cell, called a dendrite. The branching dendrites and axons enable the nerve cells to have many synapses, which is what we call the complex of the presynaptic terminal and postsynaptic density. The pores on any single postsynaptic density do not usually allow enough flow of sodium and potassium ions to cause the action potential, but if a number of them are activated, then there is enough flow of ions to activate the action potential-generating pores. A diagram of a synapse was shown in Chapter 1.

The biology may seem too simple to explain the complex processes of the brain, but several features quickly elaborate its complexity. First, there is an intriguing combination of analog and digital mechanisms. The analog mechanisms are the dendrites, which act to sum the influence of large numbers of synapses until the ion flow is sufficient to generate an action potential. Neurons have many thousands of synapses, often from thousands of other neurons. Although we do not know how information is stored by neurons, many neurobiologists believe that subtle changes in the postsynaptic density increase or decrease its response to incoming or afferent information. Analog mechanisms, which sum small differences in many afferent inputs, are extremely powerful ways to combine information. Second, the digital mechanism, the action potential, like all digital signals, has the advantage of supporting high-fidelity transmission of information, because the digital signal is either on or off. The on-off signal is quickly transmitted over the axons and can go great distances, allowing the brain to increase dramatically in size in human beings. Furthermore, axons are insulated by a fat called myelin, which does not conduct electricity, so that like a wire bundle, many axons can travel together. Finally, axons branch and the action potential travels down each branch. Thus, a neuron can have many axon terminals, called efferents, that spread its influence over many other neurons. As the axons reach the next neuron, they are called that next neuron's afferents. The convergence of many afferents onto one neuron and the divergence of a neuron's efferents to many other neurons give the system tremendous computational power. Multiplying that power by billions of neurons gives the brain its ability to process extremely complex information.

Neural Networks

Many of the converging and diverging synapses support the organization of parts of the brain, particularly the cerebral cortex, into networks. Information reverberates in the networks as one neuron excites and is excited by many others. If you are as old as I am, your brain now works slowly enough that you can catch the network in action. When you forget a name and it simply will not come to you, think of as many features of the person as you can, not only physical features but also situations or places in which you have interacted with him or her. Then turn your attention elsewhere. In about 3 to 5 minutes, while you are thinking about something altogether different, the missing name will pop strongly into your awareness. The remarkable part of the phenomenon is not that you have eventually recalled the name. Rather, what is remarkable is that the process goes on out of your awareness and then the result, the name, intrudes on what you are currently thinking. The interpretation of this phenomenon is that a reverberating network, composed of neurons that excite each other, is started into action by all of the associations that you have made to the forgotten name. Each of these associations activates a small group of neurons that in turn excites other neurons in a network. Because of the neurons exciting each other, the network increases its activity until the missing piece of information at the center of the network of all the associations is activated. Exactly how the neurons code the information is unknown and no one neuron seems to be specific to any one piece of information. Rather, the network holds large amounts of information, with activation of one bit able to influence the activity of a closely associated bit.

The synapses of the network do not all use the same neurotransmitter. There is generally a single major neurotransmitter per neuron, but there are a number of such neurotransmitters, in different types of neurons. The most common neuron, which we have been discussing, is called an excitatory neuron. Its neurotransmitter is glutamate, a very common chemical in the body, an amino acid most often used to make protein. In the postsynaptic density, however, there is more than one receptor for glutamate. The most common type of receptor responds to glutamate by opening the sodium channels, so that the dendrites become less electrically negative, moving the cell as a whole to an electrical potential that will initiate the action potential. There are over a half dozen varieties of this receptor, suggesting that it is important to nerve cells.

Inhibitory Neurons

If the nervous system had only excitatory networks, their convergent and divergent excitation would lead to every neuron discharging all the time. Not only would that lead to biological consequences such as an epileptic seizure, but also if every neuron is excited, then there is no ability to store information. In any information storage system there must be an "on" as well as an "off" condition. Therefore, in all brain areas there are neurons that have much different properties than the excitatory neurons that we have been discussing. These neurons have small dendritic trees and project their axons only to other neurons within a small area. Therefore, they are called interneurons, because they are part of the connection of neurons in a limited area. Unlike the excitatory neurons whose synapses activate other neurons, these neurons decrease the activity of other neurons. Therefore, they are called inhibitory interneurons. A typical interneuron is the basket cell. Its dendrites receive synapses from nearby excitatory neurons, so that when they are active, it becomes active. Its synapses form a basket around the axon of one of the excitatory neurons. When the basket cell discharges an action potential, it inhibits the ability of the excitatory neuron to discharge. Thus, a network containing that excitatory neuron could not be over-activated, because the inhibitory interneuron maintains control over the activity. The inhibitory interneuron uses a different neurotransmitter, gamma-amino-butyric acid (GABA). GABA opens a different kind of ion channel in the postsynaptic density, a chloride ion channel. These chloride ion channels stabilize the membrane potential at a low level so that an action potential cannot be discharged. GABA has several types of receptors, just as glutamate does. The sum of glutamate and GABA neurotransmission, one opening pore for sodium potassium and the other for chloride, determines whether the target postsynaptic neuron increases its activity if glutamate prevails, or decreases its activity if GABA prevails.

Neuronal Activity in Humans

How can we investigate neuronal function in the living human brain? The oldest tool for recording the activity of neurons in the human brain is the electroencephalogram (EEG). Small gold disks are pasted over various parts of the scalp. When ions flow across the membranes of neurons, they create an electrical field. Under some circumstances, the field is strong enough to affect the flow of electrons in the gold disks. The disks are connected to wires that lead to amplifiers, which increase the voltage 10,000-fold so that it can be processed. The simplest processing is to display the voltage change over time, the traditional EEG record. The first recording of the human EEG, using a galvanometer to capture the signal on moving paper, was performed by Erlanger and Gasser. They believed that these records would be particularly useful for understanding schizophrenia. They were perhaps the first, but certainly not the last, in their hope and belief that a particular new imaging technique would reveal the cause of schizophrenia. While the EEG can detect stages of sleep and the presence of epilepsy and other pathological features, it does not detect diagnostically significant problems in schizophrenia. It also does not detect the response of the brain to a specific piece of information, like a tone. The reason that we cannot see the response to the tone is that there are many processes ongoing in the brain. Neurons are all discharging action potentials in a cacophony of activity, from which the processing of a single stimulus cannot be extracted.

A common strategy for simplifying the neuronal voices is to perform the experiment multiple times and then average the results, linking each average to the stimulus in time. If we play a stimulus many times and record brain activity after each stimulus, then to the extent that the same circuits are activated each time, we have the same activity unfolding over a fixed time. If the electrical activity is the same each time, then it begins to sum, whereas the noise, the activity of all the other neurons in the brain that are not responding to the sound, begins to cancel out. Technically, the activity in response to the stimulus, which is the signal we wish to detect, grows as a simple sum, whereas the random activity of all other neurons, the noise, grows as the square root of its sum. After 4 trials, the signal is 4 times greater, and the noise is 2 times greater, so that the signal to noise ratio, a measure of our ability to detect the signal accurately, has doubled. After 64 trials, we have a signal multiplied by 64 and noise by 8, for a signal-to-noise ratio of 8. Somewhere between 32 and 64 trials is the minimum needed to detect the response of most brain areas to a sensory stimulus. With this strategy, we can use safe, noninvasive EEG electrodes to record the response of the brain itself to the kinds of sensory stimuli that seem to bother persons with schizophrenia. We will not be able to record the activity of individual neurons, but we will be able to record an overall level of activity from a group of neurons, identified by their response at a specific time after the stimulus occurs.

It would be desirable to examine both excitation and inhibition, the two basic electrophysiological features of the brain. If we could record the responses of neurons individually, then we could determine when excitatory neurons discharge and when inhibitory neurons discharge, but our noninvasive EEG-based techniques do not permit that level of analysis.

Sherrington's work on the inhibition in the spinal cord that we mentioned in Chapter 1 developed a strategy for examining the effects of inhibition even when the nerve cells responsible for the inhibition cannot be individually recorded. An incoming signal activates neurons through their dendrites. When these neurons discharge, they transmit activity to other excitatory neurons in their network. That is the principal means by which the brain processes information. Each neuron makes some decision about whether to discharge and transmit the signal, based on other inputs, all of which sum their activity at the dendrite. The averaged evoked potential essentially records the movement of a signal through the network. Within this network is a second kind of circuit, in its simplest form a feedback circuit. The excitatory neurons activate dendrites of a second type of neuron, called an inhibitory interneuron. As discussed earlier, it is inhibitory, because its axons release the inhibitory neurotransmitter GABA, and it is an interneuron, because its own axons will not project to neurons outside its local network. When the excitatory neuron discharges, it excites the interneuron, which feeds back the excitation to the principal neuron as inhibition, making it less likely that the principal neuron will fire in the immediate future (Figure 3-1).

A simple demonstration of sensory gating can be conducted by examining the response to two identical stimuli. In most areas of the brain, the response to the first is greater than the response to the second because the first response activates inhibitory neurons that diminish the second stimulus. As the time between the two stimuli is increased, the second response increases in amplitude until at some point it is identical to the first response. The time course from maximum decrement of response to the second stimulus to no decrement is called a recovery curve, because early neurobiologists assumed that there is a fatigue of neuronal function and that, given enough time, the nerve cells could recover from the fatigue. We now understand that the reason for the decrement is that inhibitory neurons, activated by the first stimulus, inhibit the response to the second stimulus.

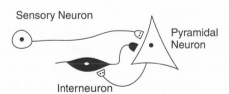

Figure 3-1. *A simple feedback circuit can inhibit the response to the second stimulus of a pair. The first stimulus activates the principle pyramidal neuron through an excitatory glutamate-mediated synapse. As the pyramidal neuron discharges, it activates the inhibitory interneuron, which in turns activates its inhibitory synapse on the pyramidal neuron. A second stimulus, delivered during the period of inhibition, then sums its activation of the excitatory synapse with the interneuron's inhibitory synapses and the response to the second stimulus is diminished.*

Gating and Neuronal Inhibition

In our laboratory, we repeat a stimulus, a click sound, at 0.5 second intervals, precisely the tick tock of a grandfather clock. To enable us to record the EEG response, we repeat the tick tocks themselves at 10-second intervals, until we have delivered 32 such pairs. Our entire experiment takes just over 10 minutes. How did we choose these times? The experiment has been used extensively in animal neurophysiology and it is well known that inhibition lasts for at least 8 seconds in the cerebral cortex. Therefore, the interval between experiments has to exceed 8 seconds. The 0.5 second was determined by varying the interval between the two stimuli to determine at what interval persons with schizophrenia have the most differences with normals. The 8- to 10-second time has a psychological concomitant that you can experience yourself. You can tap a table with a spoon, tick tock, at 10-second intervals, and record the sounds on a tape recorder. When you play it back, and wait for each pair, it will often seem like they will never come, as if somehow the tape recorder has broken. But then all of a sudden they seem to appear almost unexpectedly.

So let's look at the results of an experiment that started with a clinical observation and used a psychological theory to design a neurobiological test. The recording is called an averaged evoked potential. Averaged, because we are looking at the sum of 32 trials, divided by 32 to give us mean or averaged values. Evoked, because we used a stimulus, a sound, to detect the brain's response. We already know that this averaging technique enables us to see the response to sound by improving the signal-to-noise ratio. Potential, because what we are measuring is positive and negative electrical voltages, which are also called potentials. Normal subjects have a series of responses to the sound, with one of the more prominent potentials being positive and occurring about 50 milliseconds after the stimulus. It is therefore called P50. We picked P50 because it is less affected by the subject's interest in the stimulus than later potentials, whose amplitude depends on whether the subject's attention is directed to the stimulus.

In normal subjects, the P50 response to the first stimulus is about 5 microvolts. The response to the second stimulus is less than half that value, which is consistent with some inhibition of the second stimulus. For a person with schizophrenia, the first stimulus produces a potential that is similar in amplitude to the potential observed in the normal subject, but the response to the second stimulus is not nearly as inhibited as it was in the normal subject (Figure 3-2). This result suggests that persons with schizophrenia are missing an inhibitory function.

Is this defect responsible for their sensory gating abnormalities? It is difficult to make a leap from one level, a subjective experience, to another, a neurophysiological abnormality. If we were repairing a computer where we did not have a full circuit diagram available to us, we might run a diagnostic program to check the integrity of all the memory chips. Although we use the computer to play video games, we test it by asking each chip to memorize 1's and 0's. If one chip failed the test, then we would assume it was responsible for the computer's failure, but to test that assumption we would need to replace the chip with a functional one. To do that test, we need to find out a great deal more about inhibition of P50 responses and the failure of that function in schizophrenia. As informative as EEG recordings from the surface of the scalp might be, it would be better to examine the circuits at the single neuron level.

This paradigm has several advantages for understanding the neurobiology of schizophrenia. First, the stimuli are simple and identical, like

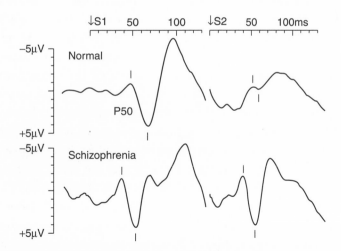

Figure 3-2. *Electroencephalographic evoked potentials recorded from the surface of the head of a normal person and a person who has schizophrenia. Both respond to the first stimulus with a P50 evoked potential. The normal person inhibits most of the response to the second stimulus, but the person with schizophrenia does not.*

the 1's and 0's in our computer diagnostic, so that we do not have to consider their interpretation by the brain, as we would have to do if the stimuli were words or pictures. Second, the patient does not have to make a response, so that we do not have to be concerned about his or her motivation. A third advantage is that we can present these stimuli to laboratory animals and record their responses. Monkeys, cats, rats, and mice also show diminished response to the second of repeated stimuli. Therefore, if we can determine the neurobiology of this inhibition in these animals, we might be able to predict how it malfunctions in schizophrenia. There is no animal model of schizophrenia, as we have discussed already, but neurobiological experiments in animals can pinpoint which neuronal mechanisms are responsible for a normal physiological behavior that we believe may be abnormal in schizophrenia. In addition, we can determine if there are interventions that reproduce the physiology that is abnormal in schizophrenia. The cardinal symptoms of schizophrenia involve the formation of thoughts that we do not believe are within the mental capability of most animals. Therefore, the analogy between a person with schizophrenia and an animal model can only be at the most elementary level of neural processing. However, we postulate, at least among mammals, that the brain is similar enough at these elementary levels to make these models useful.

A few words about the welfare of the animals are warranted. Animal modeling of human illnesses is a well-established strategy for medical research, but not one without its critics. Universities such as mine protect animals against inhumane experiments, by requiring that a veterinarian review each experiment to ensure the absence of any unnecessary pain. The animals in experiments that I will describe, mice and rats bred for laboratory use, receive an injection that induces an anesthetic state that renders them unconscious and insensitive to pain, which we verify by their absence of movement to pinch of their paw. At the conclusion of the experiment, later that same day, their brains are removed for further studies under the microscope. They die without ever having awakened from the anesthesia. Thus, they do not experience pain. However, is it right that they lose their lives in the service of our understanding more about the neurobiology of schizophrenia? Each individual who works in a laboratory weighs these decisions, as does society as a whole in its decision to permit and to fund such research. Most of us believe that if the experiment can produce worthwhile information to combat a gravely disabling human illness, then the loss of animal life is justified.

The rat brain is in many ways similar to the human brain, which makes these experiments possible. The chief difference is in the size of the brain and in the development of its cerebral cortex. Both humans and rats have a cerebral cortex, but the rat's is much smaller and not well divided into many different kinds of areas. The frontal cortex is particularly small, compared to humans. However, we know that the rat brain has all the parts that process auditory sounds from its ear up to the cerebral cortex and that these parts are nearly identical to those in humans.

Understanding the Neuronal Circuits in Animals

Now we are ready to do the experiment to discover how the brain inhibits its response to repeated stimuli. The goal is to record the electrical activity of the individual neurons, the basic unit of the nervous system, in different brain areas while the animal hears the repeated sounds. Even a small brain like the rat's contains millions of nerve cells. To narrow the search of where we want to look, we will use evoked potentials, the same technique that we used for the P50 wave described above, which records on the scalp surface. If we place a small wire on top of the rat's skull, we record a series of waves in response to the repeated sounds, just as we did in humans. There is a small wave P20 followed by a larger N40. The P20/N40 complex is decreased in response to the second stimulus, just as it is in normal humans. What we record above the skull is obviously generated by nerve cells in the brain below. The question of where exactly in the brain can be answered by moving the electrode into the brain itself, something that is occasionally done in humans, when we look for a difficult-to-treat area that is causing epilepsy, but not something that we do routinely in persons who are not ill.

In the rat we learn that the P20/N40 is largest in the hippocampus, in a region called Cornu Ammonias 3 (CA3). Part of the lore of brain anatomy is that many areas, like the seas and mountains of the surface of the moon, were named for shapes and properties that reflect the history of their discovery, rather than what we currently understand about their function. The hippocampus is a curling structure that was thought to resemble a sea horse, hence the Latin name *hippocampus*. Ammon was a neuroanatomist who dissected the hippocampus and was impressed that it resembled a curling sheep's horn, hence *cornu* or horn of Ammon. The hippocampus has five regions, labeled CA1 to 4 and the dentate, which is an undulating region that in cross-section looks tooth-like. As we move the electrode all through the brain, the P20/N40 wave peaks in size in the main layer of cells of CA3.

We now know where neuronal activity forms the P20/N40. Next, we need to know how it gets there. We know that the cochlear hair cells in the ear first generate the activity, and we can use the evoked potential technique and a knowledge of how the auditory system works to trace how information gets to the CA3 region of the hippocampus. The brain is a layered system, which reflects our evolution from the ancestor of invertebrates, a sort of primitive squid. As this primitive animal evolved, it developed some cells that could contract and cause movement, and other cells that were sensitive to features in the environment, such as touch, temperature, salt content, and light. It would be desirable when the animal were touched if it could then move in response. But that required a new kind of cell, a nerve cell, to connect the touch or sensory cells to the contracting or muscle cell. The first nerve cells were huge, clunky affairs. They moved ions back and forth, as we have earlier described, but the ion exchange moved slowly over the surface of the axon, so that the time between the initiation of the impulse by sensory activity and the contraction was long. There were times when sensation was needed to cause sudden movements and times when that was not optimal. Some nerve fibers therefore excited or activated muscle cells, while some inhibited them. The neurotransmitters that developed for excitation, glutamate, and for inhibition, GABA, at the invertebrate neuromuscular junction millions of years ago are the same excitatory and inhibitory neurotransmitters present in the human brain today. A second innovation in the invertebrate was the grouping together of neurons, so that they could begin to act among themselves to perform more complex operations. Groups of several dozen neurons could perform elementary operations, summing the input from many different sensory cells and then distributing the output to many different muscles cells. The squid's ancestors could use the neuron groups to make decisions about flight, fight, feeding, and fornication.

With vertebrates, several improvements develop in the nervous system. First, a layer of fat called myelin now surrounds each nerve fiber, which markedly improves the speed of nerve transmissions. Nerve cells can now be smaller and have more branches. And the ganglion structure of the invertebrates becomes a spinal cord and a brain. The spinal cord can handle simple reflexive, sensory, and motor coordination. The brain can then have a modulatory role, facilitating or inhibiting these reflexes. More coordinated, quicker movements than the squid was capable of are now possible with this refined nervous system. The nervous system rarely abandoned one of its older structures; rather, it built new ones on top of old ones. Fish added the cerebellum to increase muscle coordination to keep themselves swimming upright. Birds improved on the brain stem to improve visual and auditory processing. And the hippocampus appears in mammals as the first dedicated learning device. While individual synapses could change their activity based on experience, the hippocampus was a device solely interested in immediate learning. In mammals we also see the development of the cerebral neocortex, which would reach its current ultimate expression in the primates, including humans. The hippocampus is like an early minicomputer that can learn simple material, but the neocortex is more like a vast library disk storage that can store and manipulate incredible amounts of information. Rodents have some cerebral cortex, but they are predominantly hippocampal animals. They learn simple things, such as where the cat likes to hide, quite quickly, but they seem to have less capability for longer-term, more complex memories.

Information Processing in the Hippocampus

To understand the hippocampus a bit more and to decide eventually why the loss of P50 response inhibition is important, we need to understand how information arrives there.[2] Remember that the brain added layers as it evolved; it did not remake itself over for each new species. Auditory stimuli activate sensory cells in the ear, which excite the neurons that form the auditory nerve. The auditory information travels to the cochlear nucleus, which performs some rudimentary compensation for volume differences, then through the lateral lemiscus, a fiber pathway in the lateral brain stem, and on to the superior olive and the inferior colliculus. These areas, adopted from the bird brain, are important for orientation reflexes toward or away from sounds. If you hear a loud sound and turn toward it, you are using this primitive part of your brain. If you want to distinguish more, such as differences in cries associated with various mammalian animal behaviors, then you need the medial geniculate, which begins to organize the sound according to pitch, and the auditory cortex, which completes that operation. Speech perception, the highest auditory task, is entirely cortical.

Now that we have followed auditory information through its main processing centers, we can see how it comes to the hippocampus. The entorhinal cortex is part of the neocortex that is the staging area for the hippocampus. The entorhinal cortex has projections from all sensory areas, including the pathways of smell, hence its name *rhinal* or nose. The entorhinal cortex passes the information to the hippocampus via two pathways. The first pathway is to the dentate cells. The dentate is mostly composed of small cells called granule cells. The dentate was added to the hippocampus relatively late in its evolution and it gives the input a special importance, because its cells have very large excitatory synapses called the mossy fiber synapses, which have a texture in their appearance under the microscope of moss hanging from a tree. The dentate relays information into CA3 with this mossy fiber synapse. (Neuroanatomy is wonderfully descriptive and historical, but it can sometimes seem tedious to learn all the terms. Patience, dear reader, the punch line is coming.) The mossy fiber synapse ensures that the information is carried without fail to the pyramidal neurons of CA3, which will generate P20/N40 in rats or P50 in humans. In addition, however, the entorhinal cortex also sends afferent excitatory synapses directly to the CA3 pyramidal neurons via the perforant pathway, so called because it perforates or penetrates directly through the hippocampus.

The stage is now set to process information in CA3. The auditory signal arrives through a mossy fiber synapse and activates a pyramidal neuron. That pyramidal neuron activates its neighbors, which can also reactivate it. The perforant path afferents also activate the entire group. Other signals come into CA3 from other inputs and CA3 begins to form a map of the auditory and visual scene. The map is shaped by repeated reactivation from the mossy fibers and perforant pathway, which emphasize more important areas. The activity from the neighboring CA3 pyramidal neurons and their reactivation of the original activating neurons keep the image constantly refreshed. We thus have a short-term memory. If you close your eyes and then open them and are not surprised by the scene around you, it is because your hippocampus preserves the memory of where you are when your eyes are shut. Persons with schizophrenia cannot always do this simple task and sometimes suddenly feel that they are out of their bodies or in a strange new world. CA3 also acts as a "fuzzy detector." Some of its information comes not from the sounds and sights of the environment, but from the memory stores of the neocortex. Then its pyramidal activity is further enhanced and it shapes its impression of the present to determine what is new and what is not. Because the wiring is not entirely point to point, but rather depends on groups of neurons reaching the threshold for activation, the correspondence does not have to be exact. Thus, I can often recognize my wife from her walk; I do not have to check each of her features each time I see her.

If two quite important things happen near each other in time, within a half second, then I can join them in memory as one unit, either temporarily or for all time. The first short-term storage is created by CA3 neurons sending their output to CA1 pyramidal neurons. The CA3 synaptic link to CA1 neurons is capable of a phenomenon called long-term potentiation. If they are activated repeatedly and they release enough glutamate, then a special channel opens that admits calcium ions into the CA1 pyramidal neuron. The CA1 pyramidal neuron is then more easily excited for a number of minutes. This longer-term change in its activity is the first change associated with the beginning of a learning process. Here CA3's role is particularly critical. The brain's memory capacity is limited, as all of us experience from time to time. There is no way that everything we see and hear can be memorized, as Donald Broadbent realized when he was training people to identify airplanes coming across the English Channel. CA3 has to regulate the amount of information that regulates CA1 by not passing on repeated information. The reader may recognize a problem. With all this excitation going on, there would seem to be several possibilities for failure. First, we could have an explosive growth of excitation. Since all the CA3 neurons of the hippocampus form an interconnected network, then a single stimulus could cause the entire thing to become activated very quickly. That in fact can happen and CA3 is the region of the brain that is most likely to start an epileptic seizure, when it has massive discharges that cause, in turn, massive discharges throughout the brain. The afflicted person has sudden massive movements of all the muscles and then falls unconscious. There are also milder forms of hippocampal seizures, called partial complex epilepsy. In these milder forms, the person has intrusions of thoughts, often accompanied by a feeling that he or she has had the thought or experience before, called déjà vu (already seen). We can recognize this phenomenon as the manifestation of the uncontrolled activation of CA3 circuits. Sometimes the individual has this symptom when a certain sensory stimulus appears, such as a familiar tune. We can interpret this reaction as the result of the stimulus activating a very specific malfunctioning part of CA3.

Thus, CA3 is a very sophisticated part of the brain's information computer. It can do fuzzy sophisticated detection, and it sets the stage for the brain's most critical function, memory. It is particularly important in organizing information before the brain tries to memorize it. To prevent its excitatory network from running out of control, its activity is regulated by a set of inhibitory interneurons, to which we were earlier introduced. Because the interneurons sense the activity level of the pyramidal neurons and feed the information back to them as inhibition, the more the pyramidal neurons discharge, the more they are inhibited. Thus, the circuit is a self-regulation or governor of the CA3 pyramidal neuron's activity. If the interneurons are intact, the hippocampus is prevented from having a paroxysm of activity that causes a seizure. There is also feed-forward inhibition, in which interneurons are inhibited at the same time as the pyramidal neurons are activated. The perforant pathway not only contacts excitatory pyramidal neurons but also contacts the interneurons of CA3 so that it activates them as well.

Inhibition and Hippocampal Function

The interneurons' contacts to the pyramidal neurons themselves are called postsynaptic. The inhibitory interneurons sum their inhibition with the excitation of the mossy fibers from the dentate neurons, the perforant pathway synapses from the entorhinal cortex, and the excitatory synapses from other CA3 pyramidal neurons. There is a second sort of contact that inhibitory neurons make, called presynaptic inhibition. Here they form synapses on the nerve terminal that connect to the excitatory neurons, not to the nerve cell body itself, and they prevent the release of neurotransmitter from the nerve terminal. Postsynaptic inhibition decreases nerve cell activity, whereas presynaptic inhibition prevents the nerve cell from being further excited. Presynaptic inhibition works best on the excitatory connections between pyramidal neurons and on perforant pathway inputs. It does not seem to affect the mossy fibers. Therefore, the most targeted information can still reach a particular pyramidal neuron, but the spread of activity in the network is limited.

Thus, there is a second function of interneuron inhibition that presynaptic inhibition mediates. Postsynaptic inhibition prevents the network from becoming out of control, whereas presynaptic inhibition regulates how fuzzy the fuzzy detector should be. If there is little presynaptic inhibition, then there are many associations that trigger each other. If there is a great deal of inhibition, then there is little overlap between associations. There are other benefits to inhibition, however. Let's say we wanted to detect different shades of red. If we are driving and a stoplight suddenly flashes red, we want as much neuronal response as possible and slight variants in tint are not too important to us. Then an unexpected stimulus (the light turning red) encounters the network in an uninhibited state and quickly activates most of it. However, if we are looking at different shades of lipstick, then we want as much discrimination as possible. If we increase inhibition by exciting as many neurons as possible by looking at a whole counter of lipstick, then the inhibitory interneurons are also quickly excited and they inhibit the principal neurons. As a result, it becomes more difficult to excite the principal neurons and only a cell that gets the right combination of color inputs to make the perfect shade of magenta will get enough excitation to reach threshold for discharge, letting us know that we have found the right lipstick. Inhibition thus not only protects the brain from overactivation, but it also enables the brain to respond precisely when a high level of discrimination is required (Figure 3-3).

Postsynaptic inhibition is quite efficient; it works quickly and then it is over, all within 50–80 thousandths of a second. Presynaptic inhibition takes about that long to develop and then it lasts for up to several seconds and it can be extended longer, as long as the interneuron continues to discharge. Presynaptic inhibition has a time course similar to the learning of associations in CA1. The prime interval of about 300–500 thousandths of a second for learning a simple association, say between a tone and a food pellet for a rat, is the same interval during which presynaptic inhibition is most effective. When we learn a new association, we want it to be as minimally fuzzy as possible, and inhibition makes that possible.

We started talking about the diminished response to repeated stimuli as an example of sensory gating in the last chapter and now we are using

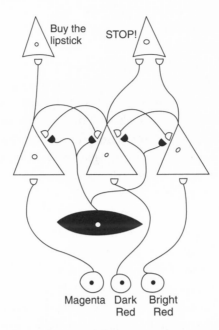

Figure 3-3. *A network of pyramidal neurons that contains an interneuron can be used to respond to all red stimuli or to respond only to magenta. When the network is first activated, the inhibitory neuron is not yet active, and any red-like color synapse activates all the neurons in the network. The network then cannot tell stoplight red from magenta lipstick. Once the interneuron is activated by the activity in the network, it uses presynaptic inhibition to decrease the release of excitatory neurotransmitter between the pyramidal neurons. Then the neurons respond only to their principal input, magenta or red. Thus, inhibition not only protects the network from runaway overactivity; it also increases its ability to discriminate.*

the paradigm to hypothesize a role for inhibition in this chapter. We have moved from the psychological world to the neurobiological world.

Persons with schizophrenia sometimes have odd associations. Remember that association was one of Bleuler's four A's. We can now understand how these odd associations arise from problems with their neural network. An example used experimentally is semantic priming. If you are asked to make the distinction between words and non-words, *church* versus *bardoc*, then your reaction time to *church* is diminished if you are primed with a preceding related word, *pew*. If the word is unrelated, *pool*, the priming effect is lessened. We conclude that *pew* is closer than *pool* to *church* in the neural network. For a person with schizophrenia, a more distant word like *death* may also prime the reaction to *church*, because there is less inhibition to retard its spread through the network. Paul confused X in his dormitory's EXIT sign with the sign of the devil. The intervening sequence was probably *cross*, *church*, *sermon*, *devil*. Loss of inhibition in the network made his thoughts freer and more dramatic, but also less well-organized than most peoples'.

4

Further Thoughts on the Fine Tuning
of Sensory Gating

As we can conclude from the previous chapter, it would be advantageous to be able to regulate sensory gating. Sometimes we want purposely to increase the inhibition to help us make the best possible judgments about what is going on around us, and sometimes it would be better to decrease the inhibition, to help us be alert or vigilant to any possibility.

The brain uses an additional set of neurotransmitters to regulate the glutamate–GABA interaction: acetylcholine, dopamine, norepinephrine, serotonin, opioids, and cannabanoids, to name a few. You may have recognized that the word *cannabanoid* is related to cannabis or marijuana. Are there marijuana neurons? The answer is a partial yes. Plants have evolved to make chemicals that can hijack our brain's carefully tuned neuronal circuits. While the human brain does not make cannabis, it does have receptors that can be activated by cannabis as well as by anandamide, which is a marijuana-like chemical that the brain does make. The marijuana plant has evolved, both naturally and now by human bioengineering, to make a compound that interacts with a human brain receptor, which is why marijuana has powerful psychological effects. Similarly, nicotine interacts with some acetylcholine receptors, LSD (lysergic acid diethylamide) interacts with serotonergic receptors, cocaine interacts with dopaminergic and noradrenergic receptors, and heroin interacts with opioid receptors. Medicinal chemists can do the same thing as plants, of course, which is why the complexity of the different chemical types of neurons is a helpful aspect of the brain's neurobiology, in terms of presenting the possibility of specific medicinal interventions to affect the activity of one class of neurons. We are going to focus on acetylcholine as a modulator of the sensory gating function. As the auditory information is on its way from the cochlear nucleus to the superior olivary nucleus, the pathway branches and some of the neurons send an axon to the nucleus of the lateral lemniscus. This nucleus projects into the brainstem reticular formation, one of the most ancient areas of the brain. It has very large neurons that are interconnected, and in many ways it is the most primitive area of the brain where neurons form a network.

Unlike the hippocampal network, which is highly interconnected and self-exciting, the brainstem reticular formation has several intrinsic limitations on its excitability. Reticular formation neurons have cell membranes that accommodate or readily stop responding after they have been activated one or two times. Therefore, the reticular formation is poor at processing the details of information, and animals whose brains are mostly reticular formation, like birds, act mostly on instinct, built-in reflexes that cannot easily adapt to new information. Scarecrows work for birds, because they do not recognize that the scarecrow never changes. Any mammal, even a mouse, quickly figures out that the scarecrows are no threat. Nevertheless, the brainstem reticular formation has an important role. It mediates startle. If a sound is unexpected and loud enough to possibly indicate a threat, then the reticular formation sends a powerful signal down the spinal cord telling the body to jump. It also sends signals forward in less dramatic cases. The signals travel to the medial septal nucleus, which is in the middle of the brain in a membrane or septum between the two halves of the brain. Here there are large neurons, which send their axons into the hippocampus in a large bundle called the fornix, which then spreads like a great tree into tiny branches or fingers called fimbria that envelop the surface of the hippocampus, particularly CA3. The cholinergic neurons of the medial septal nucleus contact many neurons in the hippocampus, but the neurons that are most heavily targeted are the interneurons of CA3 (Figure 4-1).

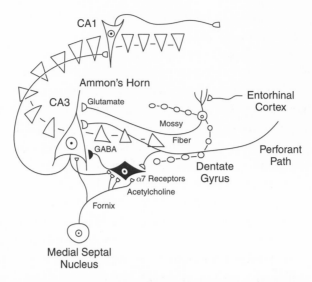

Figure 4-1. *Hippocampal pyramidal neurons and inhibitory interneurons are connected by feedback and feed-forward circuits. The interneurons are activated by acetylcholine-containing afferent axons from the medial septal nucleus. The acetylcholine that is released from these afferents activates α7-nicotinic receptors on the interneurons.*

Nicotinic Acetylcholine Receptors Regulate Inhibition

Many medial septal neurons use acetycholine, a neurotransmitter that we have not encountered before. Acetylcholine, like GABA and glutamate, is made by neurons and released onto the receptors of other neurons' dendrites and cell bodies. What makes acetylcholine interesting is that its receptors, the proteins on the postsynaptic side of the synapse, form two major families, with at least 15 different kinds of receptors between them. The cholinergic receptors were the earliest target of psychopharmacology. One family of cholinergic receptor is nicotinic, because these receptors are also activated by nicotine. Remember that abused drugs find their targets because they were developed by humans or by evolution to have specific effects on the brain's own receptors.

Nicotinic receptors form rings composed of five proteins around a hollow core or channel that is normally closed by the protein. When acetylcholine is released from the nerve terminal onto the muscle, it binds to the ring and the ring then twists open. It is sometimes likened to a lock and key. It is not only that the key fits in but also that when it does, it changes the configuration of the tumblers in the lock so that the cylinder now turns. Similarly, the core of the nicotinic receptor opens and calcium and sodium ions flow briefly into the muscle. For the muscle, the calcium ion causes the cell to contract. The protein ring then closes, with acetylcholine left on the protein. The receptor cannot then be reactivated until the acetylcholine is removed. That happens because another protein, called acetylcholinesterase, is nearby. It grabs onto the part of the acetylcholine not attached to nicotinic receptor. The acetylcholine then breaks apart and is released by both the nicotinic receptor and the acetylcholinesterase, so that both of them can participate in the activity of the next molecule of acetylcholine. The acetylcholine is actually released from the nerve terminal in small packets, the same packets that are used for its storage inside nerve cells. A whole group of packets, released at once, is necessary to admit enough calcium to produce a noticeable contraction of the muscle (Figure 4-2).

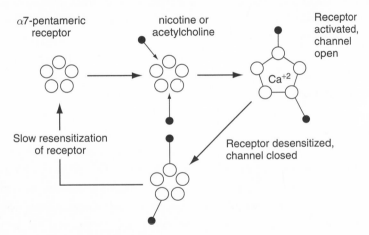

Figure 4-2. *The α7-nicotinic receptor is a five-membered ring, each member an identical α7-nicotinic receptor subunit protein. One or more molecules of acetylcholine attach to the receptor after being released from an acetylcholine-containing synapse. The ring twists open to admit calcium and other ions into the nerve cell. Then the ring closes and the acetylcholine is cleaved into fragments by the enzyme acetylcholinesterase. The receptor can then be reactivated. Nicotine works the same way to open the channel, but acetylcholinesterase cannot help cleave nicotine. Nicotine stays attached to the receptor and leaves it incapable of being reactivated. Nicotine is thus ultimately a toxin for the receptor.*

The α7-Nicotinic Acetylcholine Receptor

A similar mechanism is active in nerve cells, but the proteins in the nicotinic type acetylcholine receptor are different. The brain has a number of variants on the muscle receptor. The most common, and one even more ancient than the neuromuscular nicotinic receptor, is the α7-nicotinic acetylcholine receptor. It is more similar to the insect muscle receptor than the current human muscle receptor. It is called α7 because it was the seventh nicotinic receptor to be discovered. α1 is part of the neuromuscular receptor, and all the others are found on different types of nerve cells. It is called α because it resembles the α1 unit of the neuromuscular junction. It is located in the hippocampus on the postsynaptic surfaces of interneurons.[1] These interneurons are also the favorite target of the medial septal neurons that make acetylcholine.

Now we know the input—the medial septal nucleus neuron activity that reflects brainstem reticular formation activity—and the target, the hippocampal interneuron is responsible for focusing or unfocusing the responses of the hippocampus to sensory stimuli. We also know the neurotransmitter, acetylcholine, and its principal receptor, the α7-nicotinic receptor. We also know what the acetylcholine goes through the α7-nicotinic receptor. It opens a channel for calcium ion. The calcium ion does not make the neuron contract, like the muscle cell. Instead, it causes the nerve cell to make nitric oxide. The nitric oxide diffuses through the nerve cell and increases its release of GABA.

Now we can understand how the brainstem reticular formation helps direct attention in the hippocampus. A first stimulus arrives at the ear and travels to the hippocampus. The travel time is quick over the lemniscal pathways, through the medial geniculate nucleus, to the entorhinal cortex, and then into the dentate and its mossy fibers and CA3. The CA3 neurons respond vigorously and there is a large evoked potential summing the activity of many neurons, big enough to record its electrical activity at the surface of the head as a P50 wave. Now the feed-forward and feedback circuits in the hippocampus are activated and there is some brief postsynaptic inhibition of the hippocampal pyramidal neurons, averting a seizure. At the same time, there is activation of the reticular formation and the medial septal input, because the reticular formation has not accommodated to the new stimulus. As a result, acetylcholine is released onto hippocampal interneurons. It takes a little longer than activation through the entorhinal cortex, because the cholinergic neurons' axons are thin and do not have the myelin sheath that covers the axons of the neurons in the lateral lemniscus. Without this insulation the nerve transmits activity more slowly. However, there are fewer nerve cells in the pathway through the reticular formation, so that everything happens about the same time. The acetycholine admits calcium into the interneurons, and they release more GABA, enough GABA that now they can activate the presynaptic receptors that block the release of glutamate from excitatory nerve terminals of other CA3 neurons and of the perforant path.

At this point the hippocampus then can only be activated additionally by the more specific point-to-point wiring of the dentate granule cells and not the more diffuse inputs from the perforant path and other hippocampal pyramidal neurons. If a second stimulus occurs in the next 500 msec, the hippocampus will respond minimally, only to its most specific inputs. The response recorded at the top of the head is greatly diminished or even absent. The brain can register that a second stimulus occurred, but the highly focused minimal activity means that few resources are put to it. The first stimulus elicits, "What in the world could that be?" while the second stimulus elicits, "What exactly is that?" For example, when you walk over to the lipstick counter, the first stimulus is registered as some red color, the second as magenta.

Manipulating Acetylcholine Receptors

The rat's sensory gating can fail in a number of ways. One of the best known ways is to slice through the fimbria fornix, an experiment we obviously can only do in animals. Unlike most pathways of the brain, the fimbria fornix travels through space as a fairly distinct band between the two halves of the brain, with only fluid cavities below it. If it is cut, the animal then responds to both stimuli. We can do the same thing pharmacologically by giving a drug that blocks acetylcholine. We can be even more specific and give a drug that blocks only α7-nicotinic receptors. All three interventions lead to equal responses to both stimuli. Thus, clearly this pathway is needed and specifically the pathway needs to deliver acetylcholine to the α7-nicotinic receptor. But is it just the acetylcholine that is needed, or is the particular timing of its release also critical?

We have been painstakingly constructing a wiring diagram of the brain as if we were electrical engineers. It seems preposterous to propose that all we really need to do is to bathe the brain in acetylcholine to effect the regulation of inhibition. However, for some brain circuits that preposterous idea works just fine. The best example is the treatment of Parkinson disease. In that illness, the neurons that normally make the neurochemical dopamine are malfunctioning. Many of the drug treatments for Parkinson disease simply give a drug that works like dopamine and, at least during some stages of the illness, that is enough to restore normal movement. There is no timing of when the dopamine-like effect of the drug occurs. It is always there and it is always effective.

Could we then give acetylcholine to the animal with a sliced fimbria-fornix and restore the ability to modulate the response to stimuli? We cannot simply give acetylcholine, because the acetylcholinesterase enzyme, which is also found in the bloodstream, would destroy it before it ever reached the α7-nicotinic receptor. But there is a drug that can activate nicotinic receptors, and it is called nicotine. Let us then return to the tobacco plant to ask why it makes nicotine and what nicotine does. God probably did not place nicotinic acetycholine receptors in the brain because the Divine plan called for cigarette companies. The tobacco plant developed a toxin, nicotine, to poison animals' nicotinic acetylcholine receptors so they would not destroy the plant. The first acetylcholine receptors are found in insects, and they are the nicotinic type. Nicotinic receptors in insects, like in humans, connect nerves to muscles. In a masterful stroke of evolution, the tobacco plant has learned through millions of years to make nicotine in large amounts to combat caterpillars that would otherwise eat its leaves. When a caterpillar takes its first bite out of a tobacco leaf, it ingests a big load of nicotine. The nicotine is quite fat soluble and nervous tissue has a lot of fat in it. The nicotine therefore quickly diffuses through the caterpillar's body to the nerves that contract its muscles. The nicotine acts like acetylcholine and activates the caterpillar's muscles for one last contraction and then, because nicotine cannot be broken down by acetylcholinesterase, it stays locked onto the receptors. The receptor proteins can twist shut, so that no more sodium and calcium flow into the muscle cell, but they cannot release the nicotine. The nicotine then effectively blocks the receptor. We call this desensitization, because the receptor remains locked into a state where it cannot be sensitive to more acetylcholine.[2] The caterpillar, now paralyzed, cannot eat or breathe and falls off the tobacco plant.

Organic gardeners today use solutions of nicotine to paint on their plants to kill caterpillars. Nonorganic gardeners use a drug that blocks acetylcholinesterase, so that the caterpillar desensitizes its receptors with its own acetylcholine, which it then cannot break down. It is all the same to the caterpillar, and both compounds, nicotine and the acetylcholinesterase inhibitor, are equally dangerous to the caterpillar and to the gardener. Most nerve gases used in warfare are similar acetylcholinesterase inhibitors, as were the gases used in the Nazi concentration camps.

One of the oldest acetylcholinesterase inhibitors is physostigmine, which is a natural product from calabar beans. These were the truth beans of the Middle Ages. If an individual was suspected of falsehood, he or she was asked to eat a handful of calabar beans to see if he or she would live or die. The truthful person ate them as quickly as possible, causing a massive contraction of the stomach muscles that are also sensitive to acetylcholine, before the drug could be absorbed through the stomach lining to reach the bloodstream. The resultant vomiting purged the person of the toxic beans. The less truthful person ate more slowly, giving time for the physostigmine to be absorbed, resulting in paralysis of muscles all over the body, leading to the individual's death.

Lest this example seem too remotely medieval to you, consider another drug, succinylcholine. As the chemical name hints, it is somewhat like acetylcholine, but not quite. It also activates nicotinic receptors on the muscle and then desensitizes them. It is used during surgical procedures to paralyze muscles. Anesthetics that make patients unconscious generally do not relax their muscle tone, so that surgeons have difficulty opening the abdomen to operate. Therefore, after the patient is unconscious, the anesthesiologist administers succinylcholine. The muscles twitch and then relax. What is somewhat medieval is that the same routine is used during executions in the United States. The patient is rendered unconscious, then paralyzed with succinylcholine, and then the heartbeat is stopped with an injection of potassium chloride. The paralysis is performed not to relax the muscles for surgery, but so that the prisoner does not convulse when the potassium is administered. The execution thus appears peaceful. Some have argued that the paralysis also disguises whether the prisoner is in pain, which can also happen in surgery if the anesthesiologist does not monitor the anesthetic closely, since neither a paralyzed patient nor a prisoner can express pain by movement or expression. The debate is one more example of the influences of nicotinic pharmacology on human life.

Now we return to our animal with the sliced fimbria fornix, who is responding to all stimuli without inhibition. If we administer nicotine and stimulate with paired sounds, then the animal responds to the first sound and inhibits most of the response to the second sound. The intricate circuit that delivers acetylcholine at just the right time is in fact superfluous. Nicotinic stimulation of the α7-nicotinic receptor does quite well without it. The feed-forward and feedback circuits within the hippocampus itself are sufficient to mediate longer-lasting inhibition. Presumably the more primitive circuits of the reticular formation, which once served the purpose of calling attention to what was unexpected and possibly important, have been largely supplanted by the more sophisticated wiring of the hippocampus itself, with the α7-nicotinic receptor being the sole remnant of the older system that requires its presence.

In case you were wondering, nicotine works for persons with schizophrenia as well. "Nothing beats a cigarette," says Rachel. She says that it makes her more organized and better able to tune in to what is around her. It also decreases the voices. She does not like to smoke inside with her children around, but her backyard is scattered with ashtrays full of cigarette butts. She has a pleasant garden with several sitting places under various porches, trees, and archways, each with several overfilled ashtrays. Her mother believes that she is drinking, because she smells funny. It is stale cigarette smoke that she smells. When Rachel is in trouble, I need to meet her outside my office so that she can smoke a cigarette while her thoughts are organized. I should emphasize here that nicotine is quite dangerous, particularly when smoked and I do not advocate that patients smoke, nor do I take advantage of nicotine's quasi-therapeutic effects unless I deem it absolutely necessary. Instead, I use these insights about nicotine to help patients quit smoking, as I will outline below.

Several biographical movies of persons with schizophrenia feature smoking In *A Beautiful Mind*, Russell Crowe as Professor John Nash is first introduced to us smoking a cigarette. David Helfgott, the gifted pianist who was incarcerated in a mental hospital in *Shine*, is also a smoker. I worried when he smoked a cigarette before beginning the first movement of Rachmaninoff's Third Piano Concerto, because the

Concerto lasts longer than the time course of nicotine's effect. Sure enough, he became psychotic before the third movement.

People from around the world have written to me about smoking behavior in their relatives who have schizophrenia. One wrote that her brother smoked so heavily that the wall in his room was yellow from tar and nicotine. She said that she had learned to understand every part of the illness except this filthy habit and now she understood this aspect as well. The saddest case came in a letter from a mother who had sent her only son away to college. Tom was a young man who grew up on a farm in North Carolina. He was admitted to college, the first from his family to attend and one of the first from his impoverished rural small town. He was solitary and isolated, which is perhaps why he had time to study. Based on his grades in secondary school, he received a scholarship to engineering school and enrolled at age 17. His diary revealed that he was beginning to become suspicious of people in the college, perhaps the first signs of schizophrenia. He went to a gasoline station to purchase cigarettes, which he had somehow discovered would help him. The owner had received a citation for selling cigarettes to minors the week before and, when Tom tried to purchase them, he took no chances and called the police, who arrested Tom. Tom was released and returned to his dormitory room where, humiliated by his arrest, he committed suicide. I know that Paul could have suffered a similar fate.

In pharmacology, dose is everything and therefore we need to consider it here. The average smoker is often content with a few puffs. Smoking is the fastest way to get nicotine into the bloodstream, because the lung is essentially a huge curtain of small blood vessels exposed to the inhaled air. Just as oxygen enters the blood easily, so does warm nicotine vapor. In the next heartbeat, the nicotine is pumped from the lung to the brain. Drugs that work quickly are the most likely to be abused, because they provide instant gratification. Smoking produces effects even faster than an injection. The $\alpha 7$-nicotinic receptor is one of only 10 known nicotinic receptors. These receptors differ in their sensitivity. Receptors that contain the $\alpha 4$ unit are over 10-fold more sensitive to nicotine than $\alpha 7$-nicotinic receptors. $\alpha 4$ subunits are generally found on the nerve terminals of many different kinds of neurons and can increase the release of many other neurotransmitters, including dopamine, the neurotransmitter that is increased by cocaine. Thus, cigarettes in low doses are somewhat like stimulants, such as cocaine and amphetamine. The $\alpha 7$-nicotinic receptor requires much higher doses of nicotine for its activation. Persons with schizophrenia are rarely content with a few puffs. To get their desired effect, they need to inhale more deeply and hold their breath, giving them a characteristically exaggerated inhalation behavior that a very experienced mental health nurse once pointed out to me.

Persons with schizophrenia often have a number of odd movements, called dyskinesias, which are caused in part by the antipsychotic drugs that they take. Part of my job as a professor is to teach my resident trainees how to recognize the movements, which I do by teaching them to perform them. My rationale is that motor problems are best addressed by motor learning. An added advantage is that the resident can then show me the movement, even if the patient is not available. One of my residents came to me and told me that her patient had a movement that I had not taught them to recognize. When I asked her to show it to me, she muttered: "I knew you would make me do it!" But she complied with a series of deep inhalations with pursed lips. "I know that one," I said. "Bring him to me when he comes back next week, and I will show you what to do." She replied, "He won't stay long enough even for me to get an intake form completed. I doubt he'll stay with you." I reassured her that I was certain he would stay with me.

The next week she walked in with a grizzled veteran of the streets, reeking of many things. "I can't stay long," he said. I ran over to my assistant's office and asked for her cigarettes and a lighter. "How did you know I still smoke?" she asked. "I know," I assured her. I put the pack and lighter on the table in front of the patient, and he looked at me and then reached for them. "Thank God," he said. "I was dying for a smoke." My resident now understood his mouth movements, but her patient would not leave my office. As the office filled with smoke, I retreated and left her to fill out all the forms she wished. My assistant had gathered the entire laboratory staff outside my door. "Why are all these people here?" I asked. "I thought you were going to smoke in your office," she said. "You can get in big trouble for violating the smoking ban. I was afraid that you had cracked."

When we measure nicotine's metabolites in our patients' urine, we find that they routinely get 50% more nicotine per cigarette than other smokers, even smokers who claim to smoke the same number of packs per day. Nicotine also concentrates in the butt of the cigarette as the smoke passes through. Many persons with schizophrenia prefer butts to fresh cigarettes, because it is easier to get higher doses of nicotine from them. If the dose is raised even higher, by extremely heavy smoking, then seizures and muscle twitches result. One can also hallucinate with very high doses. Nicotine's psychogenic properties were first discovered by Native American Indians, who used it for its hallucinogenic properties at this very high dose. The hallucinations and seizures presumably come from inactivation of the α7-nicotinic receptor, which reduces the activation of inhibitory inter-neurons in the hippocampus. There is generally no paralysis from nicotine, unless someone is intentionally poisoned with it. Our neuromuscular nico-tinic receptors have changed somewhat since our caterpillar days and they are not as sensitive as the insect receptor. Our α7-nicotinic receptor on inhibitory neurons is more similar to the caterpillar's variety. That is why we can have an array of psychogenic effects, from stimulation to attention enhancement to hallucinations, with nicotine but without the paralysis. Paradoxically, the evolution in our nicotinic receptors has led to the human cultivation of the tobacco plant, precisely because we can avoid the fate of the caterpillar.

We end this chapter with the intertwining of human history, schizo-phrenia, and nicotine. What we have learned, like the sister of the patient with the yellowed wall, is that smoking is not the filthy habit of a deranged mind, but that it is a clue to a piece of neurobiology. The clue is welcome, because we have spun the story out a long way, from observations of patients in the last chapter who had difficulty with sensory filtering to an intricate wiring diagram of the hippocampus and the identification of a specific archaic nicotinic acetylcholine receptor, still with us since its evolution in the insect kingdom. The clue, the heavy smoking of our patients, never fails to remind me of two things. First, I am reminded that this neurobiological story probably has an easily observed, real-world validity, and second, I am discouraged that the current drugs we have for this illness are not doing a good enough job, because our patients like Paul have to resort to cigarettes. In the next chapter, we will test the validity of the proposition that nicotinic recep-tors are involved in schizophrenia, using an entirely different strategy. Then we will also be able to understand exactly how Paul and Rachel lost their sensory gating.

5

Insight from Genetic Studies of Schizophrenia

There is a miracle in human medical research that is unlike any other that preceded it. It is possible with modern tools of molecular genetics to discover a previously unknown biological basis for an illness simply by following its inheritance through a series of families. Then, by mapping how each person's chromosomes are inherited using the human genome map, the location of the gene variant responsible for transmission of the illness from parent to offspring can be identified. Finally, the DNA sequence of that chromosomal location can be examined to identify the variant that causes the illness. Using what we know about the DNA code, the variant's biological role can be accurately predicted and then verified. It is an entirely new strategy for medical research with enormous power, because it is independent of any previous biological hypotheses. Thus, if a disease is not well understood or, worse, if the current theories are wrong, then this method provides a fresh and often more accurate look at the problem. Muscular dystrophy, cystic fibrosis, several cancers, and Huntington disease were all solved by this new strategy in the past two decades.

For brain research, the miracle is also in the numbers. Human beings have 30,000 genes and 10 billion neurons. It seems easier to understand how 30,000 genes create the brain than to understand how the 10 billion neurons are interconnected. There are other practical advantages. It is rarely ethical to destroy even one neuron from a human being to answer an experimental question. However, the complete human genome with all the genes is present in nearly every cell of the body, including white blood cells that can be easily obtained from a routine blood sample and preserved forever as living cells in the laboratory. Also, the DNA code for genes has been deciphered and therefore their function can be understood in large part from analysis of the relevant DNA sequence. Genes are inherited by children in an orderly arrangement, based on their position on the chromosomes, and therefore an unknown gene for an illness can be deduced by observing to what extent the illness is inherited in conjunction with other known genetic illnesses nearby it on the same chromosome. We will see examples in this chapter. Finally, and most important for our investigation, the risk for schizophrenia is inherited.

As we discussed in Chapter 1, theories of the cause of schizophrenia have ranged from the theological to the psychological. The notion that a substantial part of the risk might be genetic rose to prominence in the twentieth century. The discoveries of plant genetics in the nineteenth century by Gregor Mendel, a monk who experimented with the cross breeding of peas, led to his formulation of two laws. Mendel's first law is that heritable characteristics are expressed as discrete traits and transmitted according to dominant or recessive modes. A dominant is transmitted by one parent who has the trait and one parent who does not have the trait to half their offspring. A recessive trait is transmitted from two parents who do not have the trait to one-quarter of the offspring. These patterns are easier to divine in plants, where two parents can have thousands of offspring. Nonetheless, both plants and animals have two copies of most genes and they randomly give one copy each to their siblings. Dominant traits are carried by a single genetic variant and anyone receiving a single copy of the variant has that trait, regardless of the variant that he or she received from the other parent. Brown hair is such a trait. A single copy of the brown hair gene from either parent is sufficient for an individual to have brown hair, regardless of what trait the gene from the other parent codes. Recessive traits require that both genes be the same. Thus, an offspring who receives a red hair gene from each parent will have red hair, even though both parents have one red hair gene and one brown hair gene and thus do not have red hair themselves. Most of the other offspring, on average three-quarters, will not receive two red hair genes. They will randomly receive either one or none, and thus have brown hair. Mendel's second law extends the impact of this random property: traits that are independent genetically are given randomly to each offspring. Thus, if we see two traits in a family that are randomly distributed with respect to each other, hair color and ear shape, we can conclude that they are independent genetically, whereas two that are always assorted together, red hair and freckles, we can assume arise from the same gene.

It occurred to psychiatrists at the beginning of the last century that Mendel's insights might apply to human behavior. There were large families known to be heavily affected by mental illness and developmental disabilities, some of whom were quite notorious for criminal behavior as well. One of these families in America could be traced to the immigration of a single person. An obvious solution to the issue seemed to be forced sterilization, which would prevent the transmission of these unfavorable genes to the next generation. In the United States and Europe, programs of forced sterilization were instituted as public health measures. These programs followed the most scientific principles of epidemiology, which hold that discovering the cause of an epidemic and preventing its spread are the two fundamental tools of disease prevention and eventual eradication. Ultimately, during the Holocaust, these principles were extended to incarcerate and exterminate individuals who were mentally ill. Thus, the initial application of genetics to human behavioral illnesses was not a happy one, as was mentioned in Chapter 1.

The conclusion that bad science was used to justify the Holocaust was certainly true at the end, but not at the beginning of the eugenic (good genes) movement. Much attention was given by the followers of Kraeplin in Germany to the rigorous diagnosis of mental illness, so that these traits could be distinguished by their genetically transmittable units, and to accurate population surveys, so that counts of descendants could be used to distinguish dominant and recessive patterns of heritability. Mathematical tools were developed to facilitate the analysis. Evidence that schizophrenia might be recessive—that it requires genetic contribution from both parents—was adduced. After World War II, medical scientists, in response to the horror of what the knowledge had been used for, retreated as far from genetics as possible and much of what had been learned was lost.

It is difficult, even in retrospect, to determine what principles might have been used to prevent the misapplication of the science to public policy. Certainly, we now know that the genetic knowledge was primitive, but in their day that was not obvious. We could argue that the sanctity of human life is such that it should not have been violated, regardless of the apparent scientific strength of the eugenic principles. That principle of medical ethics is called respect for persons. However, that principle carried to an extreme would prohibit all efforts of research to improve human life, since there is always risk in any research project. Eugenics did not cause the Holocaust, but it made the Holocaust more publicly acceptable than it otherwise might have been, were it solely an anti-Semitic movement. In particular, it gave a false biological validity to the concept that some people are inferior to others. That contradicts the principle of medical ethics called justice, that the burdens and benefits of research should be equal for all people. Perhaps the lesson of Holocaust science is that scientists are no better than the moral quality of the society in which they live.

Genetics returned to the fore a decade after the closing of the concentration camps to answer what had become a therapeutic question. As we know, psychological theories of schizophrenia had become prominent during the mid-twentieth century. They culminated in a series of theories that viewed schizophrenia primarily as the result of the influence of a schizophrenogenic mother. Gregory Bateson, one of the leading theorists holding this view, was a well-known anthropologist, in part because he was married to Margaret Mead, but he had no clinical background. In his theory, the mother is harshly critical and at the same time does not allow the child any independence. The child is in a double bind—he cannot please his mother and yet he cannot leave his mother. The father is passive and allows the mother to single out one of the children in particular for this treatment, who then becomes ill. Since schizophrenia does stress families, there was no problem with finding these families and discovering anecdotal evidence that fit this prediction, although there was never a rigorous test of the hypothesis. Nonetheless, the phrase stuck and it colored the relationship between these parents, psychiatrists, and even society as a whole. As Paul's mother told me, "We were the bad parents. We knew that as soon as we brought Paul for treatment that the spotlight would turn on us."

This kind of parenting problem turned out to be generally associated with ill children and not specifically associated with schizophrenia. It has been characterized in children with developmental delays leading to mental retardation, severe asthma, inflammatory bowel diseases, and juvenile-onset diabetes. In each case, the severely ill child and the family are locked together. Any stress in the family results in a flare of illness in the sick child, and the child's illness is the greatest source of stress in the family. The therapist who comes into the situation and assigns blame to either parent or child becomes a third actor in this complex drama, whose judgments increase guilt and stress. Skilled family therapists avoid placing blame while they try approaches to decrease family stress by emphasizing positive things that the family can do together that do not involve illness or control of behavior by any party.

This issue was confronted by Paul Meehl at an annual meeting of the American Psychological Association, in his groundbreaking presidential address, "Schizotaxia, Schizophrenia, and Schizotypy," already mentioned in Chapter 1. Meehl observed how many of his colleagues were engaged in family and psychotherapeutic interventions based on the idea that mothers cause schizophrenia. Meehl proposed that schizotaxia, the process that causes schizophrenia, was a genetic problem in the inhibition of excess sensory information. Schizotaxia usually caused a personality difference, which he called schizotypy, perhaps manifest as suspiciousness, timidity, and magical beliefs, but not psychosis. The psychosis of schizophrenia then occurred only in the presence of additional factors, of which the stress of an unhappy maternal–child bond was only one possibility. The scheme was a good one. It accounted for what geneticists call partial penetrance, a genetic variant producing an illness in some but not all individuals. It posited an environmental factor, which needed to be combined with the genetic variant to produce illness. Unfortunately, the definition of schizotypy, as the manifestation of schizotaxia in a normal individual, has not proved possible to implement in practice. We have no clinical test to recognize someone who is a gene carrier, although it is true that in the families of persons who have schizophrenia there are a number of people with odd ideas, including suspiciousness and magical ideas, and sometimes hypochondria.

Heritability of Schizophrenia

Extensive research with twins was used to establish that schizophrenia is a genetic illness. Monozygotic or identical twins, who come from the same fertilized egg, share all their genes, as well as most of their non-genetic influences. Dyzygotic twins or fraternal twins share two different fertilized eggs that are in the womb at the same time. Genetically, they are like other siblings and share half their genes, with the sharing of any one particular gene being entirely random. They also presumably share much the same environment, particularly if they are of the same sex, which is generally required for research. Since monozygotic twins share all their genes, they are always of the same sex. For schizophrenia, monozygotic twins have a concordance—that is, if one has schizophrenia so does the other—of about 50%. Thus, there is a significant genetic influence, since the likelihood of a person at random having schizophrenia is only about 1%. But illness is only 50% likely, which means that other, nongenetic factors must enter to cause illness. These other factors can range from prenatal nutrition, which is not always the same for the two twins because they can get different shares of the mother's placenta, to post-birth head injuries, to infections, to stress from mother and father, all of which may be somewhat different between the two twins, despite the fact that their childhood is as shared as any two persons' can be. The dizygotic twins have a similar sharing of life's ups and downs, although each has his or her own placenta. Thus, environmental factors, as important as they are, should about equalize in the two different types of twins, and the differences in genetic sharing, 100% versus 50%, should determine most of the difference between the twins. For dizygotic twins, the concordance is about 15%, less than the concordance rate for monozygotic twins of nearly 50%.

You may recognize that if schizophrenia were caused by a single genetic variant, then if the monozygotic twin rate is 50%, the dizygotic twin concordance should be half that, or 25%. The one genetic variant responsible for schizophrenia must be present in one of the parents and therefore given to each twin 50% of the time, so that if one twin has it, then the other twin has a 50% chance of also receiving it. The fact that the dizygotic twin concordance falls below 25% suggests that the single variant gene model is incorrect. If there are multiple responsible genes, then the dizygotic twin concordance quickly drops, because each gene is randomly distributed. To take the example further, if one dizygotic twin has schizophrenia caused by two independent genetic variants, then the probability that one is inherited by the second twin is 50% and the possibility that the other is inherited by that twin is also 50%. The probability that both are inherited by the second twin is 50% times 50% or 25%. Therefore, the concordance in dizygotic twins would be 25% of the 50% observed in monozygotic twins who share all their genes, or about 12%, which is what is actually observed. Thus, the twin research tells us that schizophrenia is inherited, but it also gives us the warning that the heritability will be complex. A prediction of the twin data is that the children of monozygotic twin pairs in which one has schizophrenia and the other does not should have the same rate of schizophrenia, regardless of whether their parent was the twin who had schizophrenia, which is actually observed.

Knowledge of the statistics of how schizophrenia is inherited can be quite helpful to families where there are individuals who have schizophrenia. The most frequent question comes from sisters of persons with schizophrenia, who themselves are not ill and who fear having children because they have spent much of their childhood dealing with an ill sibling and do not want to repeat the experience as mothers. For any given child their risk is 3% of having a child who will become ill, regardless of how many cases of schizophrenia are in their family. Paul's sister asked to meet me with her fiancé, who was reluctant to complete the marriage, because he also did not want to have a child with schizophrenia. I explained that we all knew her family history, but I did not know his. He told me that he had no history, because he had no living relatives. I asked how his mother had died and he explained that it was from breast cancer. I then found out that his two aunts and his grandmother had also died of breast cancer. He took his fiance's hand and with a deep sense of apology asked if she would still marry him. Today, they have two wonderful little boys. There are two points here. First, the risk of schizophrenia is about 10% from parents and siblings, the first-degree relatives, and about 3% from second- degree relatives, uncles, aunts, and grandparents. The only two high risks are monozygotic twins, about 50%, and the offspring of two parents with schizophrenia, about 40%. When I know that someone is coming for counseling about parenthood because there is schizophrenia in the family, the risk can only be about 3%, unless the partner has schizophrenia. Therefore, the important history to take is the family history of schizophrenia in the supposedly unaffected family. More likely, the partner has another common genetic illness in his or her family—cancer, diabetes, early cardiac disease, or Alzheimer disease—that is just as serious.

Heritability also becomes an issue in the case of adoption, when a mother who has schizophrenia wishes to adopt her baby. There the risk is about 10% that her child will develop the illness later in life. Adoptive families understandably differ on how they regard this risk. The demonstration that the risk for schizophrenia in children of mothers who have schizophrenia remains, even if the child is adopted by another mother close to the time of birth, was historically the most dramatic proof that schizophrenia is a heritable illness and hence a biologically based outcome, rather than a psychologically based outcome.[1] The study was performed using Danish records, because Denmark allows the cross identification of the records of adoption with the records of treatment of mental illness. The potential misuse of such records by either individuals or governments has led to a highly decentralized recording keeping system in the United States. The recently enacted federal Health Insurance Portability and Protection Act raises barriers and penalties for sharing medical records across institutions for research use. As a result, the National Institutes of Health and pharmaceutical companies under the direction of the Food and Drug Administration spend billions of dollars to perform research into disease prevalence, its response to current treatments, and the side effects of those treatments. All these studies could be better done and done more cheaply if existing data from every patient in the United States were available for research by properly qualified investigators, with a system that disguised individual identities. The Denmark system, which was used to combine two highly sensitive pieces of information, adoption and mental illness, has not had a breach of security that has harmed any individuals or their families.

The Danish adoption studies showed that the offspring of mothers with schizophrenia carry their elevated risk of schizophrenia to their new families and thus demonstrated that the risk was genetic, not the psychological stress of poor parenting. As Meehl hypothesized, the risk was for a spectrum of illness from schizophrenia itself, to brief psychotic episodes that did not develop into chronic schizophrenia to schizotypal personality disorder, in which the individual has some of the signs and symptoms, even hallucinations and delusions, but not behavior so altered as to require intervention such as hospitalization.

Some adoptive families with children who develop schizophrenia have been studied intensively and found to have more disturbed communications between parents and children than adoptive families with children who have similar putative genetic risk that do not develop schizophrenia. The suggestion is that the parenting environment still plays some role, in the context of a pre-existing genetic risk. Given our field's previous history of blaming parents for illness, one has to be quite careful in evaluating this conclusion. First, the child whose biological mother has schizophrenia and who then develops the illness is in retrospect 100% likely to have inherited the genetic risk for schizophrenia. The child who has a biological mother who has schizophrenia and who does not show signs of illness had a 50% chance of getting any particular genetic variant from her, but given that the child is not ill, one cannot say with certainty what was actually transmitted. Because there is no illness, the most likely possibility is that the child did not receive all or perhaps any of the variants that convey risk for schizophrenia. It is possible that a disturbed family environment is an additional causal factor that produced schizophrenia in the child, but it is equally possible that a child with the genetic predisposition to schizophrenia has perturbed the family's environment, particularly around the time that the schizophrenia developed.

The family's reaction to schizophrenia is different for each family. However, one of the most characteristic patterns is an organization of the family around the ill child. In many cases one or both of the parents become totally devoted to the cause of maintaining a personal interaction with the ill child, to the entire neglect of the children in the family who are not ill. In some cases, one of the parents, usually the mother, tolerates abuse of the other children—physical, verbal, or sexual—by the child who is developing schizophrenia. The abuse is recognized and justified to the other children as "he cannot help himself." A schism then often develops between the ill child and the mother and the rest of the family. I believe that the attraction to the ill child occurs because during the early stages of illness, usually in teenage years, the child remains "reachable." That is, the mother can talk to her child, and the child turns away from the psychotic ideas and can interact as her child with her. She in essence can save her child through the strength of her own love. It is a powerful emotion that I have found cannot fully be overturned by appeals to what is known about the illness or by acknowledgment of the neglect of the other children.

During his teenage years, Paul's mother was able "to bring him out of his shell." While his sister was not physically abused by Paul and in fact he was not overtly psychotic while he was at home before college, his sister recalls feeling that he used his silence and withdrawal to coax affection from her mother, in a way that she resented. Her home became uncomfortable for her, because it was centered around Paul, and she spent much of her high school years at a boyfriend's house, because he was more interested in her than her mother seemed to be. Her own psychosexual development thus began prematurely because of her brother's illness.

Because the natural history of the illness is to worsen during teenage years, the results of the parents' efforts are frequently disappointing. There is often anger at the doctors, because the child comes to treatment with anxiety and depression, the early symptoms of illness, and receives a vague, nonspecific diagnosis. Within several years, the illness has worsened despite treatment, and the diagnosis and prognosis are now more grave. Still, there are flashes of the child that once was and the mother clings to those brief moments as hope that she can reverse the illness. Parents are dismayed that the diagnosis and prognosis are worsening, despite the money and effort spent for treatment, which now seems wasted.

Amidst all these emotional interactions between parent and child is the genetics itself, the transmission of genetic variants from one generation to the next. Genes are coded for in DNA, a huge winding molecule that directs the synthesis of the proteins that create our body's structure, from its bones to its skin to its organs down to the receptors on its nerve cells. Part of the DNA has a code for sequence of amino acids, the building blocks that are strung together to make proteins. Other parts signal when and how much protein to make. Still other parts splice parts of the protein in and out as needed by the cell. We understand some of how DNA does all these jobs, but not everything. Furthermore, DNA is a fuzzy record of heritability. On the one hand, it is generally faithfully duplicated, so that genetic information is not only transmitted from parent to child, it is also transmitted from the fertilized egg to all the cells of the body, including those in the brain. However, there are occasional mistakes in the accurate duplication of DNA. If the mistake is in a cell somewhere in the body, then it may result in a growth abnormality, such as a tumor, or it may simply result in the death of that one cell. But that mistake will not be transmitted to an offspring. When mistakes are made during the formation of sperm or egg, however, then the mistakes become incorporated into the human genome and can be transmitted from parent to child and, over generations, form major variants in human beings. The uncertainty caused by the mistakes is important for human beings, because it is the mechanism of evolution. Most variants are silent; because they disrupt the many regions of DNA that apparently have little current function. Others change gene function and these can change the organism, to improve its characteristics, like increasing intelligence during the evolution of humans from the prehominids, or they can alter gene function to produce disease.

One of the uses of variation in DNA is to map illnesses to chromosomes. If there is a common variant in a particular region of DNA that is found in a family where one or more members have schizophrenia, then there is the possibility that the genetic abnormalities that cause schizophrenia are in the same area of the chromosome as the variant. Then, as we examine families with schizophrenia, we expect to see codistribution of the variant with the illness. A few families can thus indicate which chromosome contains genetic abnormalities that convey risk for schizophrenia. But chromosomes contain thousands of genes. Narrowing the field of interest to smaller regions of the chromosome takes advantage of a genetic event called recombination. During the formation of sperm and egg the two copies of almost all chromosomes pair. The exception is that the X and Y (male and female) chromosome pair in the formation of sperm. The two are then separated to form a sperm or egg that has only one copy. Fertilization restores two copies, which become the first cell of a new human being. During the pairing, the two chromosomes are very close to each other and sometimes, generally one or two times per chromosome during the formation of each sperm or egg, one chromosome breaks and joins the other, breaking it at exactly the same place. The result is a new chromosome with part of what came from the father. This process is called recombination, because the two chromosomes recombine to form a new one with parts of both.

If two genes are close together, the chance that a recombination event will occur between them is quite small. The farther they are apart, the greater the chance. Recombination can thus help assign the order of genes on chromosomes. Mapping by recombination depends on finding rare families that have recombination events near the disease-causing variant. To map to within a million or so base-pairs of DNA may require examining several thousands of offspring to find one that has a recombination with informative markers on both sides.

Genetic variants, also called polymorphisms, are detected by sequencing the DNA in the chromosome. DNA has four letters in its code, adenine (A), thymine (T), cytosine (C), and guanine (G). The DNA is analyzed chemically to determine the nucleotide base sequence (C, G, A, and T) in each person in the family. Variants can occur for a variety of reasons, but the most common appears to be a chemical alteration of the DNA by the natural processes inside the cell itself. C to T is the most common change or mutation. Depending on where in the code it occurs, the mutation can be silent or quite deleterious. Either way, these single nucleotide changes, also called polymorphisms, which mean multiple forms, make it possible to tell from which chromosome and from which parent the polymorphism came. These DNA changes likely did not occur in Rachel's family, but rather many generations ago. However, we can use them to follow the genetic transaction of illness through her family. Thus, if the common form of a sequence is CTACTC and one of the parents has CTA_TTC instead, then we can follow that region of DNA to see which offspring receive it.

Without going into the chemical details, let's say we have a test tube assay for CTACTC and CTA_TTC. One method is to bind the complementary binding sequence GATGAG to a transistor in a microcircuit. DNA is constructed like a zipper, which has one string of bases paired to another, hence the term base-pairs. G's and C's pair, and A's and T's pair. GATCAG is a perfect match to CTACTC but not to CTA_TTC. The transistor transmits a different amount of current for the two sequences, which is what we measure. In Table 5-1, we show Rachel's family. We have analyzed the DNA sequences for both members of a pair of chromosomes for each person.

Rachel, whom we have already met, has schizophrenia, but so does her brother John. We say that her father is "informative" at the CTACTC site, because his polymorphism in one chromosome allows us to distinguish it from his other chromosome. Her mother is not, because her sequences are identical. Her father appears to be transmitting risk for illness from one of his chromosome 15's. We know this because Rachel's and John's CTA_TTC sequence, which they could only have inherited from their father, appears to be associated with schizophrenia. Note that Susan and Fred do not receive this genetic variant; they receive the

Table 5-1. Rachel's Family

Mother	Father	
CTACTC...A	CTACTC...A	Chromosome 15—1st of pair
CTACTC...A	CTATTC...G	Chromosome 15—2nd of pair

Rachel	John	Susan	Fred	Peter
Schizophrenia diagnosis	*Schizophrenia diagnosis*			?
CTACTC...A	CTACTC...A	CTACTC...A	CTACTC...A	CTACTC...A
CTATTC...G	CTATTC...G	CTACTC...A	CTACTC...A	CTATTC...G

variant on the other chromosome 15. The experiment does not tell us that CTATTC is responsible for schizophrenia. It only tells us that the DNA sequences nearby might be. We might later find something we had not initially looked for. The G that occurs in the father's sequence immediately following CTACT could be a genetic variant that diminishes neuronal growth in a previously undiscovered way. The polymorphism map of the human genome is made cooperatively by all genetic researchers and applied to many different illnesses, because there is no assumption about what we are looking for.

Some caution is needed. If we have studied just this family, the probability that this could happen by chance is 0.5 for each sibling that developed schizophrenia or 0.5 times 0.5 = 0.25 for both. The usual standard of scientific proof, when only a simple test is involved, is that the probability of the result occurring by chance be less than 0.05 or 1 in 20. Therefore, this family tree would not be sufficient to establish that this genetic region is involved in the inheritance of schizophrenia. In fact, because the test could be performed many thousands of times at different gene sites, geneticists look for probabilities less than 0.00001 before concluding that a site is linked to schizophrenia. Also, Rachel's brother Peter is a problem. He carries the same allele that we have associated with schizophrenia on his second chromosome, but he does not have schizophrenia, although he is over 40 and therefore too old to develop it. Remember that even among monozygotic twins, the concordance is only 50%, and therefore we do not expect every gene carrier to have schizophrenia.

The number of families involved in current studies of the genetics of schizophrenia using these techniques is now in the thousands. The complexities are many and include accounting for different racial backgrounds, which change the relative frequency of the polymorphisms. Other problems: schizophrenia is not generally inherited from parent to child like Mendel's traits in peas, and schizophrenia does not seem to arise from a common rare gene, but instead from multiple more common genes. All of these issues introduce statistical complexities. Other common illnesses like adult-onset diabetes have the same problem. Diabetes is currently being studied in over 12,000 families. Repositories of the DNA and diagnostic information have been created for these families so that researchers do not have to recollect these samples each time that a genetic study is contemplated. Rachel's family is in a similar repository for schizophrenia.

Nonetheless, the miracle that occurred for rarer genetic illnesses—the finding of a single gene that causes the illness—has not occurred for schizophrenia. There has been a great deal of discussion among genetic researchers about why the miracle did not happen. The pessimists point out that for a common illness in which multiple genes are involved the analysis of the final genetic model requires so many families that there may not be enough to achieve statistical certainty, even if every family with schizophrenia in the world were genotyped. The optimists point out that over a dozen genes have been identified as likely candidates, with the majority of them giving positive signals in more than one independent study. It may simply be a matter of time to take the information we have and try to understand it. I understand the pessimists' concerns. If we want to use genetic research to identify the causes of schizophrenia, then we must be prepared to play by its rules and that means we have not yet discovered the answer. On the other hand, I agree with the optimists that what we have discovered can improve our understanding of schizophrenia, even if the definitive genetic model that explains how all the genetic variants interact to produce illness still eludes us.

Investigating How Genes Impact Brain Function

To try to make sense of what we have learned, we need to reconsider what our genes actually do. The molecular biologists have a mantra: DNA makes RNA makes protein. DNA for every gene exists in all cells of the body. In each cell, there are signals that activate each gene to begin a process called transcription, in which its DNA is used to make a complementary RNA, called messenger RNA. The signals that turn genes on and off are just beginning to be understood for human cells. They are proteins made in the cell by one gene that then go to another gene and bind to its DNA and cause the DNA to twist open just a little so that the process of RNA transcription can begin. A single gene may interact with dozens of these proteins, some of which promote RNA transcription and some of which repress it. Just as the nervous system performs complex operation by the interaction of excitation and inhibition, so does the biology of each cell define its structure and function by the process of gene promotion and repression. Thus, a cell with the same DNA can be a skin cell or a nerve cell or a fat cell, all by the action of repression and promotion. Cells can also respond to immediate needs by altering gene expression. For example, during stress there is release of cortisol from the adrenal gland. The cortisol enters the brain and signals proteins in neurons to begin to activate genes that will change the way that neurons respond to norepineprhine or acetylcholine, by increasing or decreasing the transcription of the RNA that makes the receptor proteins for these neurotransmitters. RNA is generally translated into proteins, because it carries the message of the gene, which is the instructions to make a precisely ordered string of the amino acids, choosing from the 21 normally found in the body. The string of amino acids is bound together to become a protein. We think of protein as muscle mass, but that is only one kind of protein. Most of the 30,000 genes make other proteins, which more often have a signaling role than a role in movement. The α7-nicotinic receptor is an example of such a protein.

The molecular biologists' mantra ends at protein, but that is where we need to extend the mantra. The genetic miracle of rare illnesses demonstrates the fact that in those illnesses a genetic error in a single protein is enough to destroy a cellular function to such a degree that an illness results. In the case of schizophrenias and other common illnesses, there has not yet been any evidence of such a dramatic loss of cellular function. As we said in Chapter 1, the brain looks pretty normal and persons with schizophrenia can do just about anything that anyone else can. Therefore, we need to think about the mantra a bit more and ask what we might expect a protein to do that would result in a contribution to the risk for schizophrenia. What we expect the protein to do is called a phenotype. A phenotype can be anything we can observe, from the level of a protein to a body characteristic like height. The closer the relationship between a gene and phenotype, the more likely we are to achieve the statistical certainty that we need to make valid conclusions from genetic research.

Figuring out the phenotype of a genetically complicated illness is not simple. The best evidence that schizophrenia itself is not a good phenotype is that in monozygotic twins there is only 50% concordance. Thus, even knowing that the twins' shared genotype can produce schizophrenia in the ill twin, the probability of the schizophrenia phenotype is only 50% in the co-twin. In more common families, we know that the probability that an offspring with schizophrenia has a parent with schizophrenia is only 10%. In other words, 90% of persons with schizophrenia do not have ill parents. We know that these parents, one or both, have conveyed genetic risk factors for schizophrenia, but the risk factors are not apparent as an illness. Meehl proposed that schizotypy was the more common outcome or phenotype of genetic risk for schizophrenia. Many researchers have tried to construct diagnostic schemes for schizotypy that would lead to its usefulness as the phenotype for schizophrenia, but so far none of these has succeeded.

For schizophrenia, genotyping is easy, but phenotyping is difficult. What we have to do is to find a function that is more closely related to a single protein than the illness itself and then see if that function—the phenotype—is linked to a single gene. At the same time, we have to make sure that there is some evidence for genetic linkage to schizophrenia; otherwise, our phenotype may have no relationship to the illness. You will notice that now we are introducing some of our biological knowledge into our investigation, which we had hoped not to do. On the other hand, we can use the genetic analysis to test whether we were right or wrong about the biology. If we are wrong, then we have genetic proof that we are wrong and we can make another choice of phenotype. Biological research into schizophrenia unaided by genetics does not have the capability of testing a hypothesis by such an independent means.

Just as we tried to unravel the neurobiology by asking what simple things persons with schizophrenia cannot do, we now ask the same question looking for a phenotype for genetics more closely related with a single gene effect. Because these phenotypes, unlike the illness itself, are not clinically apparent, they are called endophenotypes. A common medical example of an endophenotype is intestinal polyps. These polyps do not come to medical attention unless they undergo a transformation to colon cancer. Yet it is the formation of polyps, not colon cancer itself, that is inherited. For our endophenotypes, we will again turn to inhibition and excitation, the fundamental principles of the nervous system's operation and a long-recognized deficit in schizophrenia. It is quite a test of the validity of the endophenotype and the precision of its measurement, because individuals have to be declared to either have or not have a deficit, so that the pattern of deficits in a family can be compared to the pattern of genetic transmission. We phenotyped individuals several times to make sure that we saw the same results repeatedly. We constructed several preliminary studies to try to determine if the phenotype was genetically transmitted. For example, we identified families in which one parent had both an ancestral history of schizophrenia and an offspring with schizophrenia. The second parent had no such ancestral history. The first parent was therefore a putative carrier of the genetic deficits associated with schizophrenia. These first parents, but not the second parents, had deficits in auditory evoked potential inhibition that were similar in magnitude to those of their ill offspring. The loss of inhibition appeared to be a trait that might reflect the phenotype of a gene that causes risk for schizophrenia more faithfully than clinical symptoms of schizotypy.

We then performed a series of genetic studies in nine large families, each of which had multiple cases of schizophrenia in more than one generation or branch of the family.[2] Such families can generate a statistically significant probability that the association did not occur by chance. We used markers across the whole genome and found some evidence for genetic linkage to the deficit in inhibition in some of the families at markers on chromosome 15. Chromosomes have two arms that extend from a protein in the middle called the centromere. The short arm is called p and the long arm q. Under the microscope, chromosomes have distinct bands that appear when they are stained. These bands are numbered and used to help locate genes. Our statistical signal was at 15q14, or band 14 on the long arm of chromosome 15. Genetics is a wonderfully collaborative exercise, because laboratories all over the world share their knowledge of the human genome. We called investigators at the Salk Institute who had told us that they were working on the

DNA sequence of the gene for the α7-nicotinic receptor subunit, which is called *CHRNA7* (cholinergic receptor nicotinic alpha7). Once the sequence of a gene is known, part of the sequence can be made radioactive and used as a probe to attach to the specific area of the chromosome that carries the gene. Their probe attached to 15q14.

For ease of study, the human genome has been broken into small parts, each of which has been placed into a yeast colony. The small part of the human genome is carried by the yeast as an additional chromosome, called a yeast artificial chromosome. The colonies can be searched using a gene sequence as a probe to find the one that contains part or all of the gene that you wish to study. We therefore identified the yeast colony that contains *CHRNA7*. In initial gene searches, one looks for highly variant or polymorphic sequences of DNA within the gene. Some of these are single nucleotide polymorphisms, but others are repeated sequences. The most common is the repetition of the bases CA. The enzyme that helps duplicate DNA to make sperm or eggs can make rare errors, and when it gets to CA, it sometimes puts in a number of CAs before it moves on down the strand. There can easily be several dozen repeated CAs. Most often, the enzyme works correctly, so that if your mother sends you a chromosome with 14 CA repeats at a certain site, then you have 14 CA repeats in that chromosome. If your father has only 12 in the chromosome that you received from him, we can then use the number of CA repeats to determine which chromosome came from which parent. Thus, the inheritance of rare errors serves to mark each chromosome.

Families are more likely to be genetically informative using this type of genetic marker than with the single nucleotide change we examined in the example earlier. It is frustrating to spend the effort to genotype and phenotype a family only to find that they are genetically uninformative because they all have the same marker sequence at the location you want to study. As more of the human genome is sequenced, more polymorphisms are discovered which make more families informative. The CA repeat that my colleague Sherry Leonard and her research group discovered turned out to be in the second intron of *CHRNA7*. The part of the gene that codes for amino acid sequences is called its exon. *CHRNA7* has ten of them. During RNA transcription, these are spliced together to form a single messenger RNA that directs protein synthesis. Different splicing can occur from the same gene, giving rise to a family of proteins that resemble each other and yet are different in different cells. The presence of introns between the exons makes these splicing patterns. Since introns themselves do not direct protein synthesis, they generally have more variants than exons, since a variant in an exon could alter the function of the protein by changing its amino acids. Intron polymorphisms can affect gene function as well, by altering splicing, but often they do not. So far as we know, the CA repeat in intron 2 is just the remnants of an error in DNA duplication that has no known significance.

Now we have the two things we need to perform our experiment. We have genetic information on our families at many sites throughout the genome, including *CHRNA7* on chromosome 15q14, and we know two phenotypes: presence or absence of inhibition deficits and presence or absence of schizophrenia. We assessed the probability of whether the association between each genotype and the two phenotypes occurred because *CHRNA7* is linked to the phenotype, or whether the relationship could have happened by chance, just as we did in the simple example above. We found that the odds of a true link between phenotype and genotype are nearly 200,000 times more likely than a random or chance association.

The relationship for schizophrenia was also positive but not enough for certainty in a genetic analysis. Why the difference? We can decide that someone has schizophrenia with some certainty, since they generally have a lifelong history of diagnosis and treatment, but in our previous example we ignored the siblings who did not have schizophrenia. There were two reasons. First, we cannot decide with as much certainty that someone does not have and never will have schizophrenia. Some may have schizotypy, but schizotypic thinking merges into normal thinking. Ten percent of the population hears voices occasionally, including a number who believe that the people on television occasionally talk to them. Many people have magical beliefs: if I give a dollar to a street person, I believe some beneficent divinity in the universe will cause my investments to appreciate. Lifelong shyness is a trait in about 20% of the population. None of these traits are diagnostic of schizotypy, and they are not even found in all persons with schizophrenia. Rachel is gregarious and manages her investments quite conservatively, without any hint of magical thinking. But Paul is quite shy, as Saul in the Bible may have been. When it came time for Samuel to anoint him King, they had to search for him, and he was found hiding in the camp's baggage (Samuel I:10,22).

Table 5-2. Rachel's Family with P50 Inhibition Added as a Second Phenotype

Mother	Father	
P50 inhibition normal	P50 inhibition abnormal	
CTACTC...A	CTACTC...A	Chromosome 15—1st of pair
CTACTC...A	CTA_TC...G	Chromosome 15—2nd of pair

Rachel	John	Susan	Fred	Peter
Schizophrenia diagnosis	*Schizophrenia diagnosis*			
P50 abnormal	P50 abnormal	P50 normal	P50 normal	P50 abnormal
CTACTC...A	CTACTC...A	CTACTC...A	CTACTC...A	CTACTC...A
CTA_TC...G	CTA_TC...G	CTACTC...A	CTACTC...A	CTA_TC...G

Unlike schizophrenia or schizotypy, P50 inhibitory deficits can be typed in all members of the family, thus increasing the information that the family provides for tracing genes. Our family with P50 inhibition added as a second phenotype is shown in Table 5-2.

We have the same information for Rachel and John, which together gave us the probability of 0.25 that there is a chance distribution of schizophrenia in this family. That probability, the same probability as getting heads twice in a row in a coin flip, is too high for reasonable proof that we are not simply observing a chance occurrence in this family. But we have information from three more siblings to consider. Not only is one sequence, from the father's second chromosome of the chromosome 15 pair, associated with schizophrenia and P50 abnormality in Rachel and John, but the inheritance of CTACTCA from the father's first chromosome is associated with normal P50 inhibition for Susan and Fred. Peter also now comes into focus. We had ignored him in our initial analysis, but now we see that he has abnormal P50 inhibition and has the CTA_TCG. We now understand that there is a biological expression of this genetic variant that we cannot see reliably in clinical assessments, but we can see more clearly at the molecular level. Now, we can do our statistics with all the siblings accounted for. The probability of seeing this distribution of the genetic variant by chance, 0.5 multiplied five times (0.5^5) is only 0.03 (3 in 100 by chance), which is considerably lower than the 0.25 (1 in 4 by chance) if we had analyzed the family only for schizophrenia.

The convergence between the neurobiological identification of the α7-nicotinic receptor as a mechanism of sensory gating and the polymorphism in *CHRNA7* as its linkage site does not rigorously establish which variant in *CHRNA7* is responsible for genetic transmission of the P50 inhibitory deficit, nor does it rigorously establish that *CHRNA7* is the responsible gene. The variant that causes dysfunction could be in a nearby gene. However, the convergence of these two lines of evidence, neurobiology and genetics, shows the eventual utility of genetic analysis in determining which neurobiological aspects of schizophrenia are part of the inherited risk for the illness and the utility of neurobiology for explaining how genetic risk is expressed as specific brain dysfunctions that produce schizophrenia. Thus, the miracle of genetics does not fully explain schizophrenia, at least not yet, but it tells us that we are on the right track with specific neurobiological investigations, a critical piece of information that we had no way of obtaining without genetics. The experience was like going on a long road trip through back roads, when you are sure you have lost your way, and then suddenly you see the sign for Jerusalem, 20 km.

The approach that we have taken with Rachel's family has been successful in understanding the transmission of schizophrenia in many other families. However, it has not resolved the heritability pattern for everyone. More puzzling is the finding that entirely different genes appear to be responsible for the transmission of schizophrenia in different families, despite no readily discernible difference in the illness among the patients. One opinion is that studies of a handful of families are prone to more error than is estimated by the statistical techniques used to analyze genetic transmission. Accordingly, the pattern of inheritance that we have deduced may simply be a chance association of the genetic variants with the illness in a small group of people. Another opinion, which I favor, is that many different genetic variants, involving different genes, can result in schizophrenia. The neuronal machinery of the brain that handles perceptions is complex, involving many neurotransmitters and an intricate development of the nerve cells and their connections, and it could certainly fail in more than one way to produce the physiological deficits that we have found in people with schizophrenia.

Furthermore, the genes themselves contain many base-pairs of DNA and there could be different DNA variants in various families that cause even the same gene to fail. This model is called the multiple rare variant hypothesis.

To try to resolve these different models, which have been advanced not only for schizophrenia but also for other mental illnesses such as bipolar disorder and autism, there are now a number of studies that examine the DNA of thousands of normal and ill individuals, looking for variants associated with the presence of illness. Increasing automation of the chemical analysis of DNA has made this approach possible. Two recent studies using large-scale automated DNA analyses have both pinpointed the area of chromosome 15 that contains CHNRA7. CHRNA7 is in a region of chromosome 15 of about 50 to 100 genes that is flanked on both sides by repeated DNA sequences. The flanking repeated sequences are areas where the two chromosome 15s are likely to pair up before their separation to form the sperm or the egg, which will contain only one of the two chromosomes. During the pairing, the two chromosomes break and recombine with each other. Because the two flanking repeated sequences are themselves similar and close together, the recombination in rare instances may result in the small region between them being excised, so that the egg or sperm has a small deletion of this region. Then, individuals may be born (fewer than 1 in 10,000 times) without receiving a copy of CHRNA7 from one of their parents.

In studies with laboratory animals, particularly mice, a similar mechanism, accomplished through genetic engineering, is purposely used to specifically excise a gene, creating a mouse called a genetic knockout. The aim is to detect the effect of the gene by eliminating it or knocking it out of the animal's genome. Mice with CHRNA7 knockouts, either on both chromosomes or on only one chromosome, have diminished sensory gating and difficulty learning complex tasks, but of course we do not know if they have schizophrenia. In humans born without a CHRNA7 on one of their chromosomes, we have a natural experiment that duplicates the mouse experiment. The majority of these individuals with one copy of CHRNA7 have schizophrenia.[3,4] They have no family history of schizophrenia, which is consistent with their parents having two copies. Thus, a rare genetic accident seems to be resulting in the new appearance of schizophrenia in a family where it had not occurred before. Of course, the natural human experiment does not exactly duplicate the genetically engineered mouse, because more than one gene has been excised. Perhaps it is one of the 50 to 100 other genes in the small deleted region or a combination of them that it responsible. *CHRNA7* therefore may not be the responsible gene. Nonetheless, the natural experiment adds uniquely valuable evidence for the possible involvement of *CHRNA7* in the genetic transmission of schizophrenia.

Families with Schizophrenia

Rachel's mother is a kind soul, who has raised two children with schizophrenia. I have never seen her angry, despite the many stresses in her family. Rachel is the older sister and Susan, a nurse, is quite protective of her. She has understood that Rachel has limited abilities from the time they were children. As their mother has aged, Susan has started the tradition of having Christmas, Thanksgiving, and Easter at Rachel's house. Rachel often takes a nap while Susan prepares the dinner. Susan told me that it was a good way for her to make sure that Rachel and her children were included in all holiday celebrations. She feared that Rachel's children would otherwise have little contact with the family. Fred, on the other hand, is an attorney and is generally irritated with Rachel. Too much family effort, in his opinion, goes into helping Rachel with things she could do herself if she were not "lazy." When he is drunk, which happens at most family occasions, he does not mind telling her so, which leads to his shouting at her and her retreating. This range of opinions from the healthier siblings is common in families with schizophrenia.

Rachel's father is a very bright man, an engineer, who is awkward and reserved, but he made a good living as a key member of an aeronautical design team because of his ability to think beyond the current problem to see how his team's designs have to integrate with other design aspects of the aircraft. He understands the neurobiology of P50 recording and the sensory gating hypothesis. He knows that he has more trouble than others in his team concentrating in a noisy environment, but he also feels that he is the only one who does not get lost in the minutiae of the problem at hand. John, the oldest son, is quite ill with schizophrenia. He left home at age 17 to live in the street, coming home periodically, where he has a basement room. He showers and washes his clothes and then comes upstairs to eat something. Except for a few grunts at his parents, there is little social interaction. Unlike Rachel, who communicates about her symptoms, he is quite guarded. He is arrested periodically, however, for shouting bizarre threats at the police who roust him out of alleys and shop doorways at night.

Peter is a very bright man. He works as an English professor at a local community college. He is quite irritable and generally questions the value of the research and worries about its confidentiality. He is particularly concerned that his college will find out about it, because of the affiliation between the medical school and other higher education institutions in our state. For many years, he refused to participate, until his son developed schizophrenia in college, much as Paul has. His son called him one evening to say that he was hearing voices telling him to kill himself. Peter called me immediately to arrange evaluation and treatment, including research participation. His son has done well with treatment, and he was able to return to college. Peter was driving home from seeing him one rainy night when his car skidded off the road, killing him. The police declared the death accidental.

We have measured several parameters of brain structure and function in Rachel's family in addition to P50 inhibition. One of the most revealing is the size of the hippocampus, which we measured using magnetic resonance imaging. Hippocampal volumes are correlated with several learning and memory functions and are therefore a rough index of the capacity of an individual to process and learn new information. They are also quite variable between families and between individuals within families, with about the same variation in size as any other body part. Overall, the size of the hippocampus in all the family members is within the broad range of normal values, but there is still considerable difference. Rachel's father has a large hippocampus, as does Peter. Rachel's is significantly smaller, as is John's. Fred's is the same size as Rachel's. Rachel's mother and her sister Susan's are only slightly larger. We therefore have a different distribution of the trait of abnormal P50 inhibition from that of smaller hippocampus. Mendel's second law had postulated that genetically unrelated traits would be separately distributed in family members. We do not know if hippocampal size is genetically determined, but it is distributed independently of P50 inhibition and therefore it is not the same genetic trait. Rachel seems to have gotten a double hit, both her father's P50 inhibition deficit and a smaller hippocampus. Not only does she need to process more information because of her loss of a filtering capacity, but she also has less hippocampus to do it with. John has the same problem. Her father and Peter, on the other hand, have larger hippocampi. Her father is quite clear that he has poor sensory gating, but for him it has beneficial results as well. We speculate that his larger hippocampus enables him to process several streams of thought at the same time in a productive, interactive way, rather than being overwhelmed by the information. Fred also has a smaller hippocampus and further degrades its function by his intoxication, but because his sensory gating is intact, he does not become psychotic.

Schizophrenia is therefore not a single gene illness, as we have already discussed. It is the result of the co-occurrence of several genetic and probably nongenetic influences in the same individual. No single deficit, including abnormal P50 inhibition, is critical for its occurrence. *CHRNA7* is the only gene identified with schizophrenia that is a neurotransmitter receptor. *COMT,* a gene on chromosome 22, changes metabolism of dopamine. Most of the other genes are primarily developmental. We will discuss their possible roles in the chapter on schizophrenia as a developmental illness.

The human genome in many ways is a biological history of humankind. It not only reminds us of our evolutionary history, but there are also events in our history that may have been genetically determined. If we return to Saul, we find that in addition to his shyness and psychosis he has one other trait, which is responsible for his being chosen king: "and when he stood among the people, he was higher than any of the people from his shoulders and upward. And Samuel said to all the people, See ye him whom the Lord had chosen, that there is none like him among all the people?" (10:23–24).

Near *CHRNA7* on chromosome 15q14 is *FBN1,* the gene for a collagen or connective tissue molecule that helps form our bones. This gene would seem to have little to do with schizophrenia. However, people who inherit deficits in this gene are exceptionally tall. Abraham Lincoln was thought to have Marfan syndrome. Most people with schizophrenia do not have Marfan syndrome, just as most people with Marfan syndrome do not have schizophrenia, but throughout the world there have been small isolated populations in which both illnesses occur together in individuals of one generation and are transmitted together to individuals of the next generation. There are reports from African Americans, Sardinia, and modern Israel of Marfan syndrome and schizophrenia's co-occurrence and co-transmission. This co-transmission seems to be a violation of Mendel's second law, because these two independent traits should be transmitted to the next generation independently. The violation occurs because both genes are in the same chromosome 15 region. Eventually, the two genetic deficits will be split apart by a recombination of the chromosome 15 copy that carries both of them, because in fact they are caused by separate but nearby genes. Their brief existence together and co-transmission is generally observed only in small, relatively isolated populations, where there are not enough births per generation to allow recombination between two genes that are near each other. This phenomenon is called genetic drift. If we had thousands of progeny, like Mendel's pea plants, any two traits from different genes would quickly be separated.

Both of Saul's unusual traits are passed on to succeeding generations. Foot deformities are the most common manifestation of Marfan syndrome and one of Saul's grandsons had bilateral club feet: "And Jonathan, Saul's son, had a son that was lame of his feet. He was five years old when the tidings came of Saul and Jonathan out of Jezreel, and his nurse took him up, and fled: and it came to pass, as she made haste to flee, that he fell, and became lame. And his name was Mephibosheth" (Samuel II:4:4). David takes Mephisobeth into his court and appoints a guardian for him. Mephisobeth comes to believe that he will be restored to the throne of Saul: "To-day shall the house of Israel restore me the kingdom of my father" (16:3), despite the fact that he lives in a disheveled state: "he had neither dressed his feet, nor trimmed his beard, nor washed his clothes, from the day the king departed" (19:24). In the same passages, David deals with a second of Saul's relatives, Shimei, whose behavior resembles that of a mentally ill street person: "And when king David came to Bahurim, behold thence came out a man of the family of the house of Saul, Shimei....he came forth and cursed still as he came. And he cast stones at David, [saying] 'Behold, thou art taken in thy mischief, because thou art a bloody man.'" (16:5–7). "And as David and his men went by the way, Shimei went along on the hillside over against him, and cursed as he went, and threw stones at him, and cast dust" (16:13). David treats Shimei by confining him to his house in Jerusalem, from which Shimei periodically escapes.

Although any Biblical account admits multiple interpretations based on the views of the reader, this rise and fall of Saul from the perspective of 3,000 years later, in an era where molecular biology has replaced demonology, has a possible explanation in two nearby genes, *FBN1* and *CHRNA7,* one which gave him his kingdom and one which made him too disturbed to rule it.

6

Paranoid Conviction

Psychosis is more than the jumble of sensory experience created by sensory gating deficits. Psychotic thoughts and experiences become a mantra of conviction by which persons with schizophrenia lead their life. Human beings have an innate ability and desire to create a story when faced with terrifying or even potentially terrifying information. In the case of schizophrenia, the story is generally paranoid—that is, it makes the terror part of a larger, not a smaller evil. The creation of the story is not comforting in the usual sense, because it makes the situation worse, not better. This aspect of creative ability would therefore appear to have evolved as part of our brain's function for defensive purposes. The story takes small signs as warnings and makes them into a more terrible whole. The story has to account for many facts; it has to have durability and therefore the individual needs to have conviction in it. And yet it needs to be formed quickly, because its true worth is in its ability to guide future actions. These stories thus use relatively small amounts of information to form principles and convictions that outlast the sensory experiences from which they are created. Sometimes the story lasts only for a few minutes, and other times it may last a lifetime.

For persons with schizophrenia, their poorly processed sensory experiences become the basis of suspicion. What begins as suspicion becomes paranoia: coincidences become the evidence for plots and the plots become more and more elaborated. Intelligence, which early in the course of illness is a protection against the intrusion of unfiltered sensation, now becomes the fuel for these elaborations. Thus, the grandest paranoid schemes paradoxically block the rehabilitation of what should be otherwise the most treatable individuals. The affected persons' own intelligence creates strongly held beliefs that isolate them from attempts by their family and therapists to help them. How are these beliefs created and how do they gain the strength of conviction that makes them a permanent part of the personality of the person with schizophrenia?

Consistent with our proposition that these stories are part of normal human behavior and brain function, we can see the stories are often part of an attempt to rationalize or normalize a series of terrifying experiences. Although Freud's analysis of Judge Schreber is often discredited because the premise that psychosis is an attempt to ward off repugnant homosexuality is not consonant with the many people who are homosexual and not psychotic, the case introduced the idea that psychotic delusions are normalizing symptoms. By normalizing, we mean that the most obviously bizarre feature of the psychosis—the paranoid delusion—is an attempt to restore normal mental function. Thus, Judge Schreber is an example of an intelligent man who is faced with sexual feelings that he has difficulty accepting and therefore suspects that they may have come from an outside agency.

The most accessible experience of this kind of paranoia is the reaction to inexplicable current events, such as terrorism. Here the entire development of the paranoid position occurs in the public media. The response to the 9-11 attacks on New York City and Washington escalated from the targeting of a few radical dissidents in al-Qaeda to a belief, held by almost the entire country, that major Middle Eastern countries, led by Iraq, were responsible for mass terrorism and even for some to the conviction that we are involved in a millennial struggle between Christianity and Islam. Side plots include the theory that George Bush, Jr., wanted to better his father by doing what his father had dared not do—conquer Baghdad—and the symmetrical theory that Osama bin Laden, the eleventh son of a powerful man who died in an airplane crash, wanted to better his father by creating his own, more spectacular plane crashes. Both of these theories come directly from Freud's Oedipal theory that sons are innately competitive with their fathers. The military-industrial complex feared by Eisenhower in his farewell speech, the multinational oil companies, and, always, the Central Intelligence Agency are characters in almost everyone's plot. Our purpose is not to make political statements, because any or all of these explanations for the terrorists' actions and the U.S. response could be true. Our purpose is to point out that we write and read stories that try to make these situations into a coherent whole for us, much as Judge Schreber tried to comprehend his own homosexual feelings.

The Onset of Paranoid Conviction

For most persons with schizophrenia, one of the contexts of these stories is sensory flooding. Patients develop schizophrenic psychoses at the same time that they are overwhelmed by primary sensory experiences and emotional experiences that they are unable to control. For them, their loss of sensory gating, in the context of emotional distress, seems to initiate the creation of these paranoid convictions. For young men, who develop most of their symptoms in their late teens, the sensory flooding and the development of their paranoid ideas often occur in a relatively brief period of their lives, frequently a period when they are first away from home.

The transition from sensory flooding to paranoid conviction is the most dramatic and most poorly understood features of the unfolding of schizophrenia. From the personal point of view, the family observes that a young man like Paul, who previously was somewhat quiet and with-drawn, but otherwise normal, now suddenly voices ideas, usually both hallucinations and delusions, that are bizarre. These hallucinations and delusions may have been held in secret for several months, but they are still relatively recent. The patient generally finds the ideas as foreign and as implausible as everyone else.

Rachel believes that there are spaceships, parked in orbit millions of miles away, that beam thoughts to her that control every aspect of her life. The spaceships send derogatory messages, calling her a worthless drunk. They also send directions to her, which tell her to walk alone, after midnight, in dangerous parts of the city. Her fear confirms to her that she is worthless and deserving of punishment. When she was young, she drank to quiet these thoughts. Now that she is sober, she marvels at the implausibility of the voices, but she never loses her conviction in their message. The medical students who hear her story write me an angry note. "Dr. Freedman, please do not bring actresses to class." How can Rachel, with all her higher education, believe in spaceships? Rachel laughs at the situation herself. How could she, who loves Virgil and Dante, end up with Star Trek for her delusion?

What the class misses is that her conviction in the idea of the spaceships transcends her reality testing. They ask, "Do you really believe in the spaceships?" She says she does, with a laugh. That frustrates them all the more, and they ask, "Do they control your thoughts with rays?" And she replies, "Sometimes." They cannot believe it, and so one of them asks, speaking a little more slowly and a little more distinctly: "You . . . believe . . . that . . . these . . . space . . . ships . . . are . . . real?" She is used to this problem: "Yes, I do." A few other questions follow about her past, and they learn that she, like them, was a graduate student, traveled in Europe, fell in love, and made a life transition from student to writer and teacher. The question resurfaces, now from a student who seems impatient with the paradox: "You really believe that there are spaceships?"

I generally intervene here to try to separate conviction from reality testing, a point missed not only by the class but also by many people who try to decide if a person with schizophrenia believes that the voices are real. If you ask people with schizophrenia if they hear voices, they generally know exactly what you are talking about. Often, like Paul, when I first met him, they are relieved that you already understand that there is a problem. A normal person generally acts puzzled and responds, "I hear you speaking right now." Persons with schizophrenia rarely confuse hallucinations of voices or delusions of control with real sensations and forces in their lives. The class is puzzled, because in normal experience we generally assume that what we objectively know to be true and real is the source of our convictions. However, it is easy to demonstrate to our class that this assumption is not true, even for a class of medical students, who are generally well grounded in reality. I ask them, "How many of you believe that you will flunk this course?" No hands go up, because failing a class is rare in a highly selected group of medical students. That is reality, and they all know it. Besides, no one would ever admit to thinking about failure. Then I rephrase the question, "How many of you have ever had the fleeting thought that it will be difficult to pass the exam?" A few hands go up, and then a few more, when I add, "...even though you immediately put it out of your mind." Eventually, with a little coaxing, about half the class admits to occasional thoughts of failure, most of which are accompanied by stress, including sleeplessness, excess eating or drinking, anxiety, and autonomic reactions, like perspiration. Although sometimes these thoughts motivate them to study, more often the thoughts make them too anxious to study productively. Now, they begin to understand how conviction can be separated from reality.

For persons with schizophrenia, the problem now becomes clearer. Conviction and reality testing, while not seamless in normal life, are more frequently separate in their mental lives. They have more beliefs that are separate from reality, the beliefs are formed from less reliable information, and they are held more strongly. But the most striking difference is that these beliefs, though isolated from reality, are held for very long periods of time, sometimes lifelong.

The sensory gating deficit is one aspect of the problem. Because more information is arriving into the parts of the brain that form ideas, patients need to form organizing ideas more quickly. Filtering serves not only to prevent stimuli from reaching higher brain centers but also to make the most salient ideas most prominent and to suppress more random thoughts. This hierarchy is lost because of the sensory gating deficit; all ideas compete to be understood and placed into a scheme of reality.

Rachel once had to be hospitalized because Nazis were trying to break her door down. She ran into the street shouting and her neighbors called paramedics, who brought her to the hospital. In the hospital, she was initially agitated, but quickly became calm with no treatment other than a sleeping pill for the first night. She described how she had been up all night and how the Nazis kept her awake all the next day, when she tried to sleep, by banging at her door. She added, parenthetically, that the noise was as loud as the construction in the area. A home visit revealed that her tiny cottage home was sandwiched between two high-rise apartment construction sites. The Nazis, about whom she could speak calmly in the hospital, were now obviously the noise of the construction around her. Construction has been ongoing for a month and therefore we could time the onset of the stimulus and the length of time needed to form the delusion and have it intrude into her behavior.

A more typical course for the first appearance of delusions is the late adolescent onset for Paul. His Harry Potter–like delusions of snakes behind the mirror appeared over the course of a semester and gradually deepened in conviction and detail. What is noteworthy about these delusions is that the stimulus is less certain than Rachel's Nazis. The dormitory was noisy, of course, but there was no clearly distinguishable stimulus and the time course was somewhat longer. We can only speculate that a constant stream of poorly filtered sensory information from college dormitory life was the fodder for his delusion building. In some cases, even the patient recognizes that the delusion comes from poorly filtered material. Reminiscent of Judge Schreber, Paul had spent much time worrying about whether he was homosexual and, even more important, whether other people so perceived him. He had a single memory of bending over to drink from a water fountain at school, when he glanced to his side and saw the basketball coach looking at him. The coach said something to him that he could not understand, but when he thought about it, which he had done daily for the past 6 years, he believed that the coach was saying that he was "queer." Thus, the sensory experiences that become delusional beliefs can range from the trivial, in the case of the coach's inaudible remark, to the inexplicable, in the case of the snakes behind the wall, to the overwhelming, in the case of the construction noise. In all cases, however, there is misperception of the sensory experience, which we interpret as evidence of a sensory gating effect. Acknowledgment of this element by the patient is common. Paul readily admitted that he might have misunderstood the coach, and Rachel quickly realized that the Nazis' origin was pile drivers. However, this recognition did little to reduce the intensity of the delusion.

Thus, there is a second element that feeds delusions: a failure of correction. For most people, reality serves to correct misperceptions. Although stories that organize sensory experience need to be formulated quickly and held with conviction, failure to correct them with new facts would be counterproductive. Anxious medical students quickly learn to study to prevent even more anxiety. For many persons with schizophrenia, ideas are much more fixed and patients return to them over and over again.

There are many reasons why family members and physicians become tired of working with or treating a particular person with schizophrenia, but probably the most common is the enduring content of the delusions. Every stressful situation seems to begin and end with the same litany of paranoid complaints. Issues with family members long ago mastered return yet one more time, as if they have never been addressed. Frequently the physician becomes an object of the paranoia as well. Slights and miscues, remembered correctly or incorrectly, become reactivated, and appointments are cancelled in anger. An idea that may be suppressed, but never corrected, becomes the nidus around which psychopathology seems to fester and grow.

The third element is conviction. The poorly formed idea, unamenable to much correction, has conviction associated with it that seems out of proportion to its other characteristics. It pervades the patient's thoughts, seemingly driving out everything else. For most of us, there is a great deal of plasticity in our thoughts. We shift from one context to another and leave our thoughts of one subject easily behind as we turn our attention to the next. . . . or do we? Our ability to formulate a story about reality only has value while the conditions that prompted the story are present. A story about an imagined slight many years ago is the stuff of fiction, not an adaptive response to life. Yet emotionally laden stories can be quite persistent and intrude into the thoughts of even the strongest mind. Sometimes the intrusion is pathological, as in the prolonged grief that sometimes becomes depression after the loss of a loved one.

Other times, however, we value the experience of creating an intrusive, long-lasting conviction. An example is a religious conversion. Here we prize the outcome that the individuals have a profound reorientation of their thinking and that the new ideas pervade every aspect of their lives. We recognize that the individual is "born again." The ways in which religious conviction occur have a number of parallels with the formation of persistent delusions.

Conviction as a Human Process

"Sinners in the Hand of an Angry God" was the most famous sermon of Jonathan Edwards, a graduate of Yale College, and one of the leaders of the American Revivalist movement in the mid-nineteenth century.[1] This movement, one of many revivalist movements that have periodically occurred in America, was a relatively peaceful one. Its predecessor, led by Cotton Mather 100 years earlier, had resulted in the Salem witch trials and executions. Both of these were mainstream religious movements, with strong endorsement from many religious, governmental, and educational authorities. Edwards was an expert in the phenomenology of religious conversion. Here we use conversion not to mean the adoption of one religion as opposed to another, but the conversion from a life where religious belief is peripheral to one where it is central and all consuming. Edwards' sermon was designed to encourage conversion. He understood that an emotional state was critical and he used the sermon to try to create fear in the minds of his listeners.

The sermon described an image: a person's soul is likened to a spider that is held in the Hand of God over the flame of a candle. At any instant, God may let go and the soul, like the spider, is consumed by the flame. The conversion is thus initiated by fear, the strongest of the emotions and the one most likely to elicit action. This imagery, even supported by Edwards' thunder and eloquence, does not seem particularly emotionally persuasive today, although thanks to the Internet, a small, but dedicated group keeps Edwards' religious work alive. Edwards knew that his fire and brimstone preaching was not particularly persuasive to adults of his nineteenth-century church either. He quickly directed most of his conversion activities toward the young members of his congregation.

The peak period for conversion thus seems to be late adolescence, also the time when most males and a number of females develop overt psychotic disorders. It is also the peak period for conscripted military service, a time when commanders of armies worldwide have observed that young men and women are more likely to follow orders that endanger their own lives than if they are allowed to mature into full adulthood. Interviews with soldiers "in harm's way" make it clear that they feel emotionally bound to the cause of their country. Late adolescence is also the time that suicide rates begin to increase. And it is a time of romantic love and sexual attraction. Humans, like birds, bond to their mothers shortly after they are born. However, they have a second bonding period to the objects of their sexual attraction in late adolescence. Reciprocally, the peak times for psychosis in women, late adolescence for some and the postpartum period for others, are also times of bonding for them, with the bonding to infants, either naturally born or adopted, a prime example. Thus, a psychotic delusion is one of many emotionally charged decisions that young people make at a very pivotal time in their lives.

Most of these life-changing decisions are made rather quickly. Army enlistment is conducted in sales offices that resemble car dealerships, with the emphasis on signing the enlistment contract that day. Elopements, too, happen quickly, impulsively, and seem more romantic than long engagements. And religious conversion is generally conceptualized not as the outcome of a long period of study, but rather as an instant of revelation, whose significance unfolds over time. The formation of a paranoid delusion has the same character of suddenness for some patients. Harry Stack Sullivan, whose book *Schizophrenia as a Human Process*, was the inspiration for the theme and the title of this book, believed that the most ominous sign in the development of schizophrenia occurred when a young man who was quite anxious and agitated suddenly became calm with a smile on his face.[2] Sullivan believed that the emotional turmoil, which was usually over sexual identity and competence reminiscent of Schreber's homosexual concerns, was suddenly resolved by the paranoid delusion that an external agency was now in charge of the young man's life. The reason that the change was ominous was that the paranoid delusion could be unshakeable and would be in complete control of the young man's life. Sullivan, working before drug treatment was available, decided that the entire hospital ward staff—physicians, nurses, and even the cleaning crew—needed to be alert to the possibility of paranoid conversion, which could occur at any time. He taught all of them that patients could undergo paranoid conversion at any time and that all of them should be alert, as there might be a small window of opportunity to engage the patient and dissuade him from the decision. There is no record that this technique was successful, but its existence in the lore of psychoanalytic literature, akin to the deprogramming tactics used for young people who have joined religious cults today, is evidence for the puzzling suddenness of conversion in young people.

Although most conversions—romantic, religious, vocational, or paranoid—are conceptualized as long lasting, we actually have little data or even observation of how long such conversions actually persist. Love deepens over time for some, but the divorce rate is high, particularly for marriages between young people. Religions have to preach to their own converts to prevent backsliding. Paranoid delusions do last in schizophrenia, but there is some evolution of content, suggesting some persistence and some formation of new delusions. In general, life's experience eventually tempers conversions and middle age brings with it skepticism of youth's passions.

The neurobiology that underlies this conversion and delusion is not clear. Clearly, it is an aspect of learning and memory, but it involves learning that occurs over a longer time course than a single experimental session. Persons with schizophrenia fall into two groups for learning and memory. One group is moderately impaired, with overall intelligence placing them in the lowest quarter of persons. They are impaired in two ways. They have poor ability to learn quickly and accurately in an experimental setting, as when they are asked to memorize lists of related words or to retell a detailed story. They also have a poor fund of knowledge about common items, like the names of animals, suggesting the effects of a chronic learning problem.

One such patient was presented to me by a resident class. I was a bit suspicious myself when this pleasant appearing middle-aged woman announced to me, when I asked her why she had come to the clinic, "I am the Queen of England." She said it blandly, without affect. The paranoid side of me wondered if the class had contrived to put one over on me on the first day of the term. How could I decide if she was delusional or if she was part of a hoax? We were in the classroom of the hospital and behind her was a map of the world and there was England in the center of it. I asked the woman to show me where on the map England was. She had no idea. I watched her eyes. She did not even glance at England. One or two more questions established that she had no knowledge at all about England. My own paranoia subsided. The delusion was the sad construction of a woman with rather limited mental abilities, which she used to place herself in a world that she barely comprehended. I then became more interested in how she dealt with this limitation in her daily life. Her routine was quite fixed, a subsistence life that took advantage of social workers, food stamps, well-known bus routes, and tolerant neighbors. Being the Queen of England meant there was little she had to explain to others and insulated her from their questions that she would have difficulty answering.

About two-thirds of patients with schizophrenia have some variant of learning dysfunction. In older diagnostic terms they were termed simple schizophrenics, a diagnostic term that disappeared because it seemed to merge with mental retardation. Some of these individuals would have inappropriate smiles, and they were termed hebephrenic, a term that has also disappeared. Neuroleptic medications commonly used in schizophrenia seem to prevent the inappropriate smiling, perhaps because it retards smiling itself. It was always recognized that there is a second group, about one-third of persons with schizophrenia, who do not have deteriorated mental functioning. This group is paranoid. The content of their thought, reflective of their intelligence, is better formed and tells us more about how the mind can go awry in schizophrenia than unfortunate patients like the Queen of England.

Perhaps the best examples of this type are very bright persons with schizophrenia like Professor John Nash, who won the Nobel Prize in Economics for his explication of what is now called the Nash equilibrium.[3] The equilibrium describes how individuals competing for the same goal establish patterns of cooperation that enable them to compete as individuals more effectively than if they pursued their individual efforts in isolation. Professor Nash's illness occurred a bit later in life than the typical adolescent onset in males, which is typical of brighter people, but it otherwise had all the well-known features of schizophrenia. Specifically, the hallucinations and delusions arose in a specific period of his life, in his case in graduate school. Although they were continuously elaborated throughout his adulthood, the basic archetypes were established in his early adulthood. The book and film about his life nicely portray his ability to see patterns in the world around him, like the Nash equilibrium. In the film, he is asked to solve a repeating code, a series of numbers in his intelligence work during World War II. For most individuals, the repetition of the numbers hides the occasional periods of information contained in their sequence. But John Nash was able to discern within the otherwise nonsensical repetitions a series of numbers that he could then interpret as longitudes and latitudes of cities, the coded information that was being transmitted to spies. At the same time, however, he sees a figure in his peripheral vision, as depicted in the film, who becomes an imagined master spy in his future delusions. Like Paul and the coach who said something indistinguishable, the man in the shadow becomes instantly fixed and prominent in Professor Nash's mental life. In obedience to orders from this master spy, he attempts to find patterns of secret communication everywhere, including his wife's magazines and newspapers. The significance of the bizarre behavior occurrence in Professor Nash's life is that low intelligence or a general learning deficiency is not the cause. Rather, the delusion arises from the same creative process that produced a Nobel Prize–winning insight.

Professor Nash is committed to the cause of research in schizophrenia, not because of his own situation, but because his son had the onset of schizophrenia in late adolescence. He does not have Nash's unusual abilities, and his situation is more grave. This unfortunate occurrence tells us that the pathological process that gave rise to the illness in the Nash family is probably the same as that which causes schizophrenia in many other people.

Professors Nash and Arthur Schopenhauer, whom we met in the first chapter, raise a critical question for us. Are their delusions simply the result of a powerful mind that makes even more powerful nonsense from a sensory gating abnormality, or do they have another pathology super-imposed on the sensory gating problem? One strategy to dissect pathologies is to take advantage of the genetic basis of schizophrenia. We bemoaned earlier that schizophrenia is a multigenic illness, with different genes of small effect contributing modestly to the genetic transmission of risk. However, its complexity is amenable to analysis using Mendel's second law, which states that traits from different genes are each distributed independently from parents to offspring. In other words, if sensory gating abnormalities come from one gene or set of genes and the abnormalities that cause delusions occur in other genes, then we should be able to observe that sensory gating disturbances occur independently of delusions in some family members.

Rachel's family and members of other families who have sensory gating abnormality, but do not have schizophrenia, might be expected to have some variant of schizophrenia. Indeed, some do. They have schizotypal personality traits, which include both positive and negative features of schizophrenia, including magical and paranoid beliefs, reminiscent of the hallucinations and illusions of schizophrenia, and social withdrawal and isolation, reminiscent of the negative features. What is remarkable is that although they have these features that seem to place them on the brink of schizophrenia, their mental health is quite stable. Although they have their share of life's problems, they do not develop schizophrenia. They appear to have problems in sensory gating but they are able to perform most frontal lobe functions, called executive functions, normally. Thus, despite the stream of sensory information that comes from their sensory gating deficit, they can generally decide what the excess information means to them and they handle it appropriately. Other siblings with sensory gating abnormalities show no overt schizotypical traits. They lead normal lives, often with considerable success. Lawyers, policemen, a few psychiatrists, and teachers are frequent occupations in our experience among siblings who have sensory gating abnormalities. These individuals provide evidence that Professor Nash's schizophrenia is not simply the result of a sensory gating deficit superimposed on high intelligence.

There are several possibilities for the production of delusions in someone like Professor Nash or Rachel. One possibility is that there is accelerated learning ability, or alternatively, diminished forgetting. There is some evidence for either or both possibilities. Here we are at one of the frontiers of neuroscience, because little is known about the mechanisms of learning and forgetting, particularly in human beings. However, pathological conditions sometimes enable medical investigators to see aspects of normal functioning that are not otherwise easy to investigate. One of the areas of the brain in which a neurobiological mechanism of learning has been identified is in the hippocampus. In our earlier sensory gating model, we examined the CA3 region, where patterns are formed. In the simplest model of hippocampal function, this area is a staging area for information that will be delivered to the CA1 region. The CA1 region is one of the brain's best identified memory areas. Animals with CA1 lesions have difficulty learning to identify signals that reward their behavior in experimental situations. A few human beings with small cerebrovascular strokes that include only CA1 have been identified. They have profound learning and memory deficits, specifically for the acquisition of new information.

The rat hippocampus has been studied in the most detail, because slices of it that contain CA1 and CA3 connected together can be removed and placed under a microscope for detailed electrophysiological recording. A single electrical pulse delivered through an electrode placed in the axon fiber tract leaving CA3 for CA1 results in the activation of CA1 neurons. The effect is quite reproducible, with the same electrical current always producing the same level of activation. The current causes impulses to travel down axons from CA3 neurons to synapses on CA1 neurons. Release of neurotransmitter from the synapses onto CA1 neurons causes them to be excited. If, instead of a single pulse, we stimulate the fibers with a rapid train of pulses, then a change occurs. Following the train of pulses, there is an enhanced effect when we return to single pulses. Each single pulse produces a larger activation. The phenomenon is termed long-term potentiation, because it lasts many minutes after the train of stimuli. We do not know what kind of learning, if any, this physiological effect mediates. One thought is that patterns of information repeated together somehow reinforce each others' importance. However, the presumption is that enhanced neuronal activation in CA1 is one mechanism that enables it to accomplish its learning function.

The neurotransmitter at the synapse between CA3 and CA1 is glutamate. As we learned earlier, a single neurotransmitter can have different functions depending on its receptor. CA1 receptors for glutmate are of a number of different types. For fast signaling between neurons, glutamate uses receptors called kainate receptors, because this function of glutamate can be mimicked by the chemical kainic acid. There is a second type of glutamate receptor on the same neurons, called an N-methyl-D-aspartate receptor, named for a chemical that mimics this function of glutamate. We have mentioned this receptor briefly before. Kainate receptors are connected to channels in the nerve cell membrane. When glutamate contacts the receptors, it opens the channel briefly to allow sodium to flow into nerve cells, resulting in brief activation. The N-methyl-D-aspartate receptor is normally blocked by an ion of magnesium, so that it cannot be opened. However, when the kainate channels are repeatedly activated, the membrane potential falls and then the magnesium ion pops out. At this point, glutamate then activates the N-methyl-D-aspartate channel. This channel opens for a longer period of time than the kainate channel and it opens wider, which allows bigger ions such as calcium ion to enter the nerve cell. Calcium ion has a longer-lasting effect, because it causes activation of biochemical processes within the nerve cell called phosphorylation. Phosphate ions are added to chemicals inside the cells, increasing and decreasing their function. Long-term potentiation in CA1 is blocked if the N-methyl-D-aspartate receptors for glutamate are chemically disabled.[4]

Glutamate receptors cannot be studied directly during life in persons with schizophrenia, but they can be identified after death in hippocampal tissue. Each of the receptor types is a distinct protein and for each protein an antibody can be made by injecting a piece of the protein into a rabbit. The rabbit recognizes it as a foreign protein and makes that antibody against it. The antibody is then obtained from the rabbit's serum and used to mark the protein in the hippocampus. Persons with schizophrenia have increased numbers of N-methyl-D-aspartate glutamate receptors and decreased numbers of kainate receptors. Thus, relative to other persons, they would have increased long-term potentiation. And so it is possible that for some persons with schizophrenia, learning through this mechanism might occur more easily.

There is some evidence for and some against the possibility of this mechanism in schizophrenia. In favor of the possibility is the finding that several of the genes associated with N-methyl-D-aspartate neurotransmission appear to be genetically associated with schizophrenia. Against the possibility is the observation that one of chemicals that disables the N-methyl-D-aspartate mechanism is phencyclidine or angel dust, a substance that itself can cause hallucinations and delusions.[5]

The hypothesis of accelerated learning has never been formally tested in schizophrenia. For most persons with schizophrenia, it probably does not occur. Instead, it is their slower and less efficient learning that contributes to their illness. For those in whom accelerated learning may occur, it is observable in their achievement before the onset of illness, but generally less so thereafter. Excess entry of calcium into neurons can be toxic to them and could account for the small but accelerated loss of neural tissue in some persons with schizophrenia.

But accelerated learning in schizophrenia can account for only a minority of cases, because the majority is clearly learning disabled. There is, however, another psychosis in which accelerated learning may play a role. In many cases of the manic phase of bipolar disorder, there is the sudden onset of rather well-elaborated delusions.

Winston was a sophomore in college, who had a brief depressive episode during which he lost interest in his studies and thought transiently about dying. He told his parents about his desperation and they brought him to the hospital. He seemed to respond well to antidepressant treatment and he was discharged. One week later, his father and his uncle carried him into the emergency department tied to a lawn chair. Over several days, Winson had stopped sleeping and had become increasingly expansive. He had announced plans to start his own college and to travel to Africa. He then for the first time experienced voices in his head telling him to jump off the top of his parents' apartment building and kill himself. He started to act on the voices, and his father and uncle then tackled him, tied him to a chair, and brought him back to the hospital.

What was remarkable about Winston was that a set of fully formed hallucinations appeared immediately, in someone of above average intelligence. The slow development of Paul's delusion of the snakes over an entire academic term was short-circuited for Winston. The content may not have been as detailed for Winston, but it was well enough formed to capture his belief and to compel him to action. One of the neurotransmitters that increases during a manic period is norepinephrine and it is one of the neurotransmitters that is also capable of accelerating long-term potentiation. Whether norepinephrine's enhancement of long-term potentiation is responsible for the rapid increase in the development of psychotic symptoms is unknown.

There is one other aspect to the mechanisms of psychosis concerned with learning that has puzzled observers. Next to nicotine, marijuana has become the preferred drug of abuse among schizophrenics. Like most drugs of abuse, marijuana is abused because it mimics an existing neuro-chemical in the brain and uses its receptors. For marijuana, these receptors are called cannabanoid receptors. Chemicals that disable these receptors exist. One of the functions that is disrupted when cannabanoid receptors are disabled is called extinction.[6] What is learned can also be unlearned. For example, if an animal hears a tone and receives a shock, it quickly learns to freeze when it hears the tone. If the tone is played repeatedly without the shock, soon the animal stops freezing in response to the tone. Its response is said to be extinguished. Just as the inhibition of sensory gating was once thought to represent a fatigue of neuronal function, extinction was also once thought to be a decay of the memory trace. The evidence that decay is not the mechanism comes the next day. If the animal, which has already extinguished its response to the tone the previous day, now hears the tone again, it again freezes. This time, if the tone is repeated without the shock, the animal extinguishes its freezing behavior much more quickly. However, the fact that the animal froze to the first few tones meant that it had not forgotten the original meaning of the tone. Instead, it had learned a second meaning of the tone, one that was less threatening. If cannabanoid receptors are disabled chemically, the extinction process is blocked. Excessive use of marijuana decreases learning functions, perhaps by increasing extinction. At any rate, just as schizo-phrenics find nicotine transiently helpful, they also report transient relief from marijuana, perhaps because of nicotine's ability to enhance sensory gating and because of marijuana's ability to enhance extinction.

The neurobiological view of schizophrenia presented in this chapter and the last is not one of deficit; rather for many patients it is one of enhancement of brain function, albeit increasingly beyond their control. The time of maximum symptom appearance then is not so mysterious. The expression of schizophrenia in late adolescence and early adulthood comes at the time of maximum mental (and physical) energy and achievement. Learning, including religious conversion, is more intense during this period than at any other time. Unfortunately, the process goes awry and the patients sense it. The loss of control is expressed by many patients. Indeed, the poignant question "Am I losing my mind?" is one that is not infrequently asked by a person who is in the early stages of schizophrenia.

7

Treatment of Schizophrenia

One might suppose that the treatment of schizophrenia arises from a fundamental understanding of its neurobiology and its psychology. However, the treatments, both pharmacological and psychotherapeutic, were not developed in this way. For many illnesses, treatments were discovered by observation of unintended therapeutic effects of medications given to patients for entirely different purposes. These medications themselves then become insights into the pathophysiology of the illness. We learned in the first chapter that such serendipitous observation of the effects of chlorpromazine led to its introduction into clinical practice and to the dopamine theory of schizophrenia. The neurobiology of sensory gating and nicotinic receptors is just beginning to prompt new experimental therapeutic development. Psychotherapeutic treatment has also been surprisingly removed from any fundamental theory of the psychology of schizophrenia. For the most part, psychotherapeutic approaches have reflected the psychotherapies currently in vogue. Psychoanalysis, which was developed for neuroses, and cognitive-behavioral therapy, which was developed for depression, have both been invoked as therapies for schizophrenia.

The treatment goals for schizophrenia are ambitious, because the disruption in brain function is considerable. Left untreated, the grip of the illness constricts the thinking and functioning of its victim. Paradoxically, both patient and family are frustrated that so much remains intact that it seems that the illness is volitional. Family members like Rachel's brother and Paul's mother wish that their relative would "just snap out of it." A second paradox is that medication is clearly the most powerful tool in treatment; yet the outcome varies widely in different psychosocial treatment settings around the world. Treatment is generally targeted in two broad ways: symptomatic relief and reversal of the decline that results from the progression of the illness.

Symptoms and Symptom Relief

Much of the work on treatment of symptoms involves attempts to improve three different domains. They are conceptualized as positive symptoms, negative symptoms, and cognitive deficits. Positive symptoms are the classic symptoms of hallucinations, delusions, and other disorders in thinking, such as confusing a part for a whole, that are termed formal thought disorder, literally a disorder in the form of thought. Rachel, for example, thought of Nazis because she had heard loud knocking and she had read of Nazis knocking loudly at the door of people destined for the concentration camp. These and other symptoms are thus aspects of mental function that are clearly abnormal in schizophrenia.

The negative symptoms are the relative absence of normal brain function. These range from inability to pay attention to avolition, the failure of goal-directed behavior, and anhedonia, the failure to have a sense of pleasure. One of the most unusual negative symptoms is poverty in the content of thought, which is best demonstrated as alogia. Alogia is absence of content of speech, even when normal speech fluency is preserved. Many persons with schizophrenia have fascinating, elaborately rich paranoid delusions that spill out of them, and immediately label them as mentally ill. For the patient with alogia the illness is not nearly as obvious. Speech has no pressure or urgency. Each question from the physician is met with a brief answer, usually a single word that invites no reply. The conversation rapidly drops to trivialities about the weather. "Fine." "Who bought the nice tie for you?" "My sister." Or even mirror speech, "Who bought yours?" It becomes maddening for the interviewer. The individual seems normal, with reasonable engagement and fluency, but he is unable to add content to the discourse. It is like speaking to a mannequin. Paul's conversation, unless he is in a crisis, is devoid of spontaneous content and emotion.

One of the most striking of all schizophrenia symptoms is an extension of alogia, the patient's terror that his thoughts have been forcibly removed by an external agency. This symptom is a good example of the blurring of the boundary between positive and negative symptoms, because this symptom can be recorded as a paranoid delusion or as the negative symptom of thought withdrawal. The German psychiatrist Kurt Schneider considered it the most pathognomonic symptom of schizophrenia. What is remarkable about the symptom is that the person himself recognizes that he has lost his thoughts. Such self-insight is less common in Alzheimer disease or other dementias, where the loss in brain function occurs slowly. Here, in schizophrenia, it appears rapidly and the patient is terrified by it. The complaint "they are taking my thoughts" may not occur exclusively in schizophrenia, but it is more typical of this psychosis than of any other. Paul's interaction with the snakes, left untreated, was progressing to this endpoint.

The third domain of symptoms is still being defined, but it is broadly termed neurocognition, a direct measure of the brain's thinking. It rises not from observation of clinical symptoms, but from clinical neuropsychology, a branch of psychology that uses standardized tests to determine the level of functioning of the brain. The tests are ranked into subdomains, such as attention, which might be measured by a single repetitive task, such as the Digit Vigilance Test. In this test, which requires that the subject cross off all the 7's in line after line of random digits, the demand of any individual action is low, but a sustained effort without interruption is required. Thus, performance of the test correlates with sensory gating abnormalities presumably because a failure of sensory gating leads to the intrusion of distracting stimuli. A second subdomain is verbal learning. Most tests in this subdomain are related to the California Verbal Learning Test. The test assays the ability to learn lists of words, some of which are related and some not. A third subdomain is delayed recall or long-term learning. Here there are differing results. In the experimental situation, a delay means a period of 30 to 90 minutes, during which the subject is engaged in other tasks. On this measurement, patients with schizophrenia usually perform well.

Attention is an example of a deficit in the cognitive domain that cuts across the boundaries of positive, negative, and cognitive symptoms. It is directly measured by a neuropsychological test and rated as a negative symptom. However, many investigators have proposed that hallucinations and delusions are the direct result of the same intrusion of sensory information that diminishes the ability to maintain sustained attention.

The reason for examining the overlap between the domains is twofold. First, it is currently believed that the domains are differentially affected by current drug treatments, with positive symptoms the most affected, negative symptoms intermediately affected, and cognitive symptoms the least so. Positive symptoms in isolation sometimes occur after medical treatments. An example is the effect of L-dopa, the medicine used to treat Parkinson disease. About 30% of patients with Parkinson disease treated with L-dopa develop auditory hallucinations. These generally vary in intensity from intrusive thoughts and words to the sensation that people are whispering or talking about them. They rarely cause a change in behavior, and the patient is relieved when he is told that the experience is a side effect of the medication. Thus, the positive symptom, by itself, is managed with reassurance.

Another piece of evidence that supports differences between the symptoms is the relationship of the various domains to psychosocial outcome. One can argue that the relative inability to form and nurture social relationships such as a marriage and the inability to obtain meaningful, long-term employment are the most significant results of having schizophrenia. Several analyses suggest that these disabilities are more closely related to neuropsychological measures of cognitive disturbance than to ratings of the positive symptoms of schizophrenia.[1]

Social psychiatry, the study of mentally ill individuals in the context of their families and their community, also sheds light on the nature of symptoms. Families in particular are quite tolerant of individuals who hallucinate and are moderately delusional. What they do not tolerate and become openly critical of is the lack of will that is the most perplexing negative symptom of schizophrenia. The patient's inability to sustain effort leading to some meaningful employment or other social role is seen as willful by families and is deeply resented, whereas hallucinations and delusions are understood and accepted as illness. Paradoxically, they accept the most bizarre features of the illness and resent the most commonplace, which they ascribe to laziness.

Thus, the three symptom domains form separate treatment targets for schizophrenia, both because they have some independence in their presentation and because they have different impacts on the patient's role in society.

The goal of treatment is unfortunately not the mechanism of treatment. If the treatment is pharmacological, then the mechanism is a neurobiological change. If the treatment is psychotherapeutic, then the mechanism is emotional and psychoeducational and involves a defined interaction between therapist and patient, and perhaps his or her family. Neither of these treatment mechanisms maps clearly onto the three domains of symptoms. It is therefore not surprising to learn that no one has ever designed a successful treatment specifically for schizophrenia. The drug treatments are based on the accidental discovery of the role of dopaminergic, serotonergic, and perhaps cholinergic mechanisms. The psychotherapies, including psychodynamic psychotherapy, cognitive-behavioral therapy, and various family interventions, were all designed for other mental illnesses and then applied to schizophrenia. There has never been a focused program of research based on neurobiological hypotheses to develop new treatments for schizophrenia. As you will realize from the previous chapters, a biological hypothesis for the illness is just beginning to emerge and to develop to the point of identifying molecular targets that can in turn be the targets for drug development.

Does Treatment Change the Course of Schizophrenia?

The antipsychotic drugs' unprecedented effectiveness for decreasing the acute symptoms of schizophrenia engendered considerable hope that the decline in psychosocial and cognitive functioning that characterized schizophrenia as dementia praecox would also be eliminated. Living among thousands of people with mental illness in a large institution, often called the back wards of the state mental hospitals, without the mental stimulation of normal life might be as responsible for the decline in function as the illness itself. Aggressive, early treatment of the illness might therefore also entirely alter the course of the illness. For example, the partial responses—diminishment but not elimination of hallucinations and delusion—that were initially observed with chlorpromazine might be more complete if the treatment were delivered before the hallucinations and delusions became chronic. Although this hope for a course-altering effect of medication may seem unique to the psychopharmacologists and biological psychiatrists, the psychoanalyst Harry Stack Sullivan had the same hope for his early intervention before the onset of chronic paranoia.

For psychopharmacologists, aggressive treatment means higher dose. As drug companies developed more specific antagonists of the dopamine D2 receptor than the original drug chlorpromazine, many, but not all, side effects were eliminated. In particular, sedation and low blood pressure, which limited the dose of chlorpromazine were much less problematic for drugs such as trifluoperazine or fluphenazine. These drugs could then be given in very high doses, to attempt to eliminate all signs of psychosis. Drugs were given intravenously in large doses as well, effectively loading the body of the patient with the drug to achieve high levels almost immediately. Neither of these strategies was effective in shortening the course of the initial psychotic episode nor in preventing the chronic phase of the illness.

What was effective was a strategy that involved the injection of a chemically altered form of the drug into the muscle. The chemical alteration, technically an esterification, means that the drug has to undergo an initial chemical metabolism to remove the added ester before it can be absorbed into the bloodstream. This process occurs slowly and therefore the drug is slowly absorbed over several weeks from the muscle into the blood and ultimately the brain. The strategy, called depot injection because the muscle injection acts as a reservoir or depot for the drug, has the advantage that it does not rely on the patient's taking the drug every day. Patients, like all of us, are better at remembering to keep an appointment for an injection than at remembering to take daily doses of a drug. Depot injection, when combined with a vigorous program of rehabilitation that aimed at finding patients a social and vocational niche, helped many patients avoid a pattern of repeated re-hospitalization.[2] The outcome was not as good with regular oral medication, even though the antipsychotic drug molecule was identical, and it was not as good if the rehabilitation was omitted. Unfortunately, depot medication also resulted in increase in some of the side effects, particular the Parkinson disease–like side effects, because of the prolonged, continuous blockade of dopamine D2 receptors.

A family practitioner called me because a 54-year-old woman had come to see him as a new patient to receive an injection of a depot antipsychotic drug, fluphenazine decanoate. Fluphenazine is a very specific dopamine D2 antagonist, related to chlorpromazine but with improved potency and specificity. The decanoate is the ester addition. He noticed that she had board-like rigidity and a fixed facial state, in other words the symptoms of early, but severe Parkinson disease. The doctor was disturbed by her appearance and referred her to me.

She told me that she had come from New York to live with her son and his young family. Previously, she had lived alone in the Bronx, where she was quite isolated and frightened by the deterioration of her neighborhood. She had received the injections for 7 years. She did not notice the rigidity. Parkinsonian symptoms are caused by blockade of dopamine in the basal ganglia, an area of the brain that operates out of our general awareness. Patients generally need someone else to tell them that they look rigid, because they are not aware of it. The family doctor was the first person to alert her to it. She told me that her psychiatrist in New York had told her to seek continuation of the injections from a family doctor, because he feared that most psychiatrists in Denver would not agree to continue them. She has not been hospitalized for psychosis during the 7 years that she had been treated with the injections. Over the past several decades, she had been hospitalized only briefly, generally several days every 2 to 3 years because her voices would begin to torment her.

I called her son and told him that I thought she should be on a lower dose of an oral medication, because she had developed the Parkinsonian symptoms and because she was doing so well. He was angry: "What's the chance she will become sick again?" I told him that I could not be sure, but his mother would be less rigid and the chances were good that she would not have a relapse that required more than a few days hospitalization, as before. He explained the problem to me: "I convinced my wife that we could have her move here, because she had not been sick for so many years. We need someone to watch our children every day, because we both need to work. If you fiddle with her medications and make her sick, I am shipping her back to the Bronx." I asked that patient what she wanted to do and she said, "I would rather be a grandmother here than go back to the Bronx. Please do not change my medication."

What I learned from the grandmother is the meaning of the interaction between successful prevention of relapse, in this case with the help of depot medication, and the establishment of a social and vocational role. She demonstrates why the administration of the medication and the social-vocational therapies have intersecting effects. Residual symptoms of schizophrenia, including side effects of treatment like Parkinsonian symptoms, are problematic, of course, but when a patient avoids hospitalization, she ceases to be regarded as a patient and becomes a person who can be relied upon and who can have a niche in her family or community. My colleague Richard Warner points out that the niche is related to the economy.[3] If the economy is booming and workers are in short supply, niches are easier to come by. In a recession, people with mental illness may have a harder time finding their niche. Therefore, when I prescribe medication I have three aims that I try to fulfill: *(1)* to achieve as much acute symptom relief as possible, *(2)* to do as much as possible to prevent relapse, and, of course, *(3)* to provide treatment that is as safe as possible given our first two aims.

The beneficial effects of preventing relapse thus provide a benefit that extends for a longer time than we might expect from the incomplete effects of antipsychotic drugs on the acute symptoms of schizophrenia. The benefit adds to the natural course of the illness for many patients. During the initial episodes, the psychotic symptoms are problematic and there are frequent relapses because of increasing intensity of hallucinations and delusions, which can often lead to irrational behavior. Sometime at the end of the first decade of illness, the intensity of the symptoms begins to decrease. I have never been certain whether the decreasing intensity results from the patient's aging, which tends to diminish the effect of catecholamines on nerve cells. Or perhaps it reflects maturity, which enables them to adhere more closely to the treatment and to be wiser themselves about how to deal with their situation. Regardless of the reason, a number of patients develop remarkable insights about themselves and find solutions in their lives that maximize their strengths and buffer them against stress that would exacerbate their illness.

I often counsel parents and patients, after we have seen initial resolution of the psychosis, that they need to expect a bumpy and discouraging decade. Frequently, as observed by Sullivan, there is complete resolution of the psychosis, and the patient can return to school or work. However, there is often a subsequent relapse, and, after several such episodes, the illness becomes chronic and a significant decline in function occurs. Paul seemed very close to becoming an engineer when he entered college, but the possibility of his finishing school became increasingly unrealistic as his ability to concentrate seemed to worsen over the first couple of years of his illness. However, as the initial decade of illness comes to an end, there is often improvement, imperceptible at first, but increasingly the patient becomes more sociable and better able to participate in life around him. Paul would develop a business and a family over the course of the second decade of his illness.

Some patients experience a more complete remission. Sarah was always a reluctant patient. Her sister had been severely ill since age 14 with schizophrenia and by age 18 was placed in a nursing home, the successor of the state mental hospitals, for custodial care that would last her lifetime. Sarah needed to distance herself. She refused to visit her sister in the nursing home, and she left Colorado for college in Boston. I met with her one Christmas vacation, because she became curious about the research that we were doing with her family. Sarah felt that if university researchers were interested in her family, she might at least find out about what they were finding. We recorded her sensory gating physiology, which was abnormal, and told her that the "test" was in fact not a medical test, but that we would be available to her in the future if she needed us. Two years later we heard from her mother that she had become psychotic. Sarah was treated at the student mental health clinic of the university that she attended and made a full recovery after 6 months.

We did not see Sarah for 10 years. She graduated from college and earned a masters degree in fine arts. She was angry, had difficulty forming stable relationships with men, and had changed teaching jobs every several years. However, there was no sign of psychosis. Twenty years after her psychotic illness, Sarah came through town again. She visited her sister briefly and came to me for advice about care for her father, who was developing Alzheimer disease. She had two children and a stable marriage and owned an art gallery. She was flamboyant, but not sexually provocative. She spoke with loud phrases and sweeping gestures in a dramatic, sometimes histrionic manner, but she was logical at all times. She had little to say about her sister, but she had much to say about her difficulties with her mother, who had a very different, but also difficult personality style. Sarah was into macrobiotic diets, and her mother was similarly attracted to low-impact organic farming. Both of them felt that the food industry either did not care about nutrition or was engaged in a conspiracy to addict people to sugar and fat. Sarah lived in a commune where there was open sharing of food, living space, and child care. Her mother had many cats and was reluctant to let anyone into her home. These extreme personality styles, which often include paranoia, are common in the families of people with schizophrenia, along with the schizotypal personality disorder that we discussed in the previous chapter on paranoid conviction.

The frequency of remission, either after a single episode or after several episodes, is unknown. Estimates range from about 10% to as high as 40% for patients who were hospitalized for an initial episode of psychosis. For some patients, continued treatment with medication is important to prevent relapse, which would destroy their psychosocial gains. Our grandmother from the Bronx probably needed her medication, and Paul and Rachel certainly did, but Sarah did not. Therefore, it is not clear to what extent the progress in the second decade is the result of good treatment and to what extent it reflects the natural course of the illness. Remissions were observed before the introduction of antipsychotic medications, but many patients remained in back wards. I do not believe that Paul and Rachel would be doing as well in the community without drug treatment. Rachel might have been sheltered by her family, because of her children, but there is a good chance that Paul would be in a state hospital.

Patients often ascribe their improvement to their psychiatrist's acumen with medication. They view the first decade as a constant switching of medications, as they and their psychiatrists struggle to find a solution that provides effective treatment and avoids side effects. With each relapse, medications are changed and doses are increased. New drugs, despite their increased expense, are tried, because one can always hope that they offer a benefit, when the older drugs do not seem to be as effective as needed. During the second decade, doses can frequently be reduced. Both Paul and Rachel take half the dose of medication that they used earlier in their illness. Of course, the side effects are much more tolerable as a result of these lower doses. Many patients are on newer drugs, because a newer drug was the latest one tried when they entered into this period of remission. It is difficult to show that newer drugs, other than clozapine, are more effective than older drugs, despite their hoped-for benefits. Therefore, public mental health systems and private insurers frequently ask patients to use the older, less expensive drugs. The cost of the drugs can represent 80% or more of the entire cost of treatment, which severely impacts the funds available for hospital care and for psychiatrists, psychologists, social workers, and case managers involved in the patients' treatment and rehabilitation. The patients and their families respond that it took a decade until Dr. Freedman got the medication "right," and they do not want to repeat that trial-and-error odyssey. While I like to be known as the doctor who got it right, in fact it is the natural course of the illness that is the reason for my apparent success.

Thus, medication has a positive, but not a curative effect on schizophrenia. Could medications be found that would have a more profound therapeutic impact? That would require intervention before the illness has become fully apparent, a topic that we will discuss in Chapter 10.

Early Treatments for Schizophrenia

The first antipsychotic drug to be discovered was chlorpromazine, as we discussed in Chapter 1. Chlorpromazine was almost immediately marketed worldwide. There were social forces both advocating and resisting its use. First, mental hospitals themselves were brutal institutions, because of their large size and the number of patients whose behavior was difficult to control. In the United States, Dorothea Dix led the first reforms in the nineteenth century which included new policies that forbid chaining patients to walls. A bell was forged from some of those chains and it is now the symbol for the National Mental Health Association. Nonetheless, straightjackets and restraints were commonly used to subdue patients. Patients were also packed in cold, wet sheets, which were thought to be calming.

Like these various forms of restraint, the "biological" attempts to control behavior also seem quite primitive in retrospect and added to the quick embrace of drugs when they became available. Observations that patients improved their mood after epileptic seizures led to therapies that induced convulsions, such as electroconvulsive therapy, in which alternating electric currents are applied to the surface of the head. The alternating current, similar to the 60-cycle current used in household electrical outlets, induces waves of excitation that overwhelm the brain's inhibitory circuits and cause seizures. This treatment, given under anesthesia with assurance of good oxygenation of the brain during the seizure, is safe, but it is effective only in limited doses for severe depression. It therefore remains in use today for treatment of patients whose depression is resistant to medications. Convulsive therapies are not usually effective for schizophrenia. When it was the only treatment available, it was given repeatedly, in large amounts, to patients with many different kinds of diagnoses, including patients with schizophrenia, but its overuse could lead to brain damage, which gave the treatment a poor reputation.

Another treatment in common use was frontal lobotomy, the surgical severing of the connections of the frontal lobe with the thalamus. This treatment was based on a neurobiological theory that reverberating circuits between the frontal lobe and the rest of the brain were responsible for obsessive thoughts, including hallucinations and delusions. Evidence of docility in aggressive monkeys who received the operation and evidence from persons who had received injuries to the frontal lobe suggested that the treatment might help control mental illness. Edgar Moniz was awarded the Nobel Prize in 1936 for the development of the treatment. It did make some aggressive patients more tractable, but at the expense of a considerable loss of their cognitive abilities. Since the treatment was expensive because of the requirement for surgery, it was first used for intractable patients whose families could afford treatment.

One of my own teachers remembered the Yale Department of Psychiatry faculty deciding to recommend lobotomy for one of their colleague's wives, when he asked his colleagues what could be done to help her with intolerable obsessions. The prospect of preventive uses was even raised, and for awhile the treatment was advocated for rebellious, but otherwise normal teenagers, with the rationale that it would prevent the onset of more serious illness. The surgery, which was first attempted by only the most skilled neurosurgeons because of the requirement for discrete lesions deep in the brain, was gradually simplified in a number of ways, with the last simplification being the introduction of a needle through the thin bone of the upper orbit of the eye into the brain and then moving it back and forth to sever the connection of the frontal lobe above. Electroconvulsive therapy was used to induce paralysis and amnesia for the procedure. It then could be performed by many physicians in mental hospitals, without the need for neurosurgeons. This chapter of psychiatry's history always sobers me, because much of the thinking—the neurobiological model, evidence from animals and humans, therapeutic enthusiasm for treatment of both the refractory patient and preventive efforts in a possible prodromal patient—are not so removed in time and in scope from our own efforts today. For many years, frontal lobotomy remained the only treatment of mental illness based on a biological theory.

The history of frontal lobotomy should remain—and is recounted here—as an object lesson for how we can mislead ourselves into harming those whom we wish to treat.[4] All biological treatments now undergo far more rigorous testing of their efficacy and side effects, and physicians are much more alert to the continuous monitoring of both these aspects of new and existing therapies, to make sure that treatments are truly beneficial. Clinical trials in which both clinical rater and patient do not know whether the treatment is a new experimental drug, an established standard drug, or placebo—termed a double-blind, placebo-controlled trial—are required. The study that led to the cessation of frontal lobotomy was such a study that included sham operations and double-blind ratings to produce definitive evidence that the lobotomy was ineffective, although the study occurred after the introduction of chlorpromazine, which had already made the operation superfluous.

Support for treatment with new medications also came from the tenor of the civil rights movements of the late 1950s. The French Revolution was the first political movement that called for emptying the mental hospitals on the grounds that hospitalization was a type of incarceration for holding unpopular beliefs. If one could be hospitalized for a paranoid delusion, then the belief that a current political regime is evil could also be labeled as paranoid and lead to political imprisonment. Such abuse is alleged to have occurred in the Soviet Union, for example. There was also a serious movement in the United States to declare schizophrenia a false diagnosis, imposed on one group of people by another. As a result in this country, the conditions for involuntary hospitalization must be strictly met, which primarily involve direct evidence, usually the patient's threat that he or she is immediately going to harm himself or another person, because of a clearly apparent mental illness. All decisions are made by judges on the recommendation of psychiatrists, with the patient represented by his or her own attorney. Even during times of crisis when it seems likely that mentally ill individuals might be confused with political prisoners, there is generally a distinction made between the two. In fact, the French quickly re-hospitalized their mentally ill patients. The Iraqi prisoners of the military forces in Abu Ghraib prison identified the severely mentally ill among themselves, arranged for their segregation from the rest of the population, and called them to the attention of U.S. medical personnel for immediate treatment.

The Success of Non-Drug Treatments

Thus, the goals of more humane treatment, the evidence for the lack of efficacy and severe toxicity of other biological treatments, and the desire to release people from mental hospitals for treatment in their own communities all led many psychiatrists to advocate for the immediate use of neuroleptic drugs. But there were also forces heavily involved in non-drug treatments that resisted the widespread adoption of medications. Various treatment facilities and programs for schizophrenia had been developed, most notably the moral treatment movement in England, which advocated placing patients into small cottages with therapeutic counselors to help them return to sanity. Groups of occupational therapists in mental hospitals in the United States found that patients were often capable of improvement and helped many of them return to their families.[5] Although some of these groups achieved remarkable success, good outcomes were sporadic and generally related to the charismatic presence of a few individual leaders. The majority of patients appeared to do well in these enriched therapeutic milieus, but they rarely left the treatment environment to resume life outside its confines.

The concept of a therapeutic environment was not a new one. From the time of the Middle Ages in Europe, the Belgium town of Gheel provided rooms in homes for persons with schizophrenia. Most of these communities provided tasks that persons with schizophrenia could do and regulated alcohol consumption carefully. The World Health Organization funded research that purported to show that schizophrenia had a lower prevalence in less developed countries, presumably because in these countries there was more need for labor and therefore persons with schizophrenia could find a role. Rural Ireland has been held to be a haven for persons with schizophrenia, who were left behind in isolation in small villages when their healthier relatives emigrated to the Americas because of the potato famine. Undoubtedly, while there are pockets of persons who have been well treated without medication, overall the outcome has not been successful. The most definitive test of drug-free treatment in the United States was performed at the National Institute of Health's Clinical Research Center in Bethesda, Maryland. Patients were hospitalized for a year in the Center during their first episode of psychosis. All of them did as well without medication as a comparable group in a community hospital who received medication. However, one year after discharge, patients in both groups were being treated in their community with medication.

The most academically powerful group advocating for drug-free therapy were psychoanalysts. Although Freud had been interested in schizophrenia, he had not advocated for psychoanalysis as a treatment for it. However, psychoanalysis itself was considered a tool for investigation, and some analysts tried it with persons who had schizophrenia under this rubric. As with all treatments, there was some success. One of the most successful analysts taking this approach was Harry Stack Sullivan, whose books on this treatment, including *Schizophrenia as a Human Process,* were so inspiring to me. Lore passed down during my psychiatry experience at Harvard Medical School told of a medical student some years before who had sat down with a patient in an acute psychotic episode and said to him, "I can see you are a very unhappy person." Reportedly, the patient responded to this empathic statement with a discussion of his problems that turned out to be therapeutic, and he left the hospital shortly thereafter free of psychosis.

During my own rotation through the inpatient service at Massachusetts Mental Health Center, a young physics graduate student was hospitalized with an acute psychosis. His professors called the hospital and begged us not to use any treatment that might destroy his mind. Therefore, he was not treated with medication for a week or so, and it was suggested that I sit with him to see if I could understand what was troubling him. He took one look at me and said, "You're the medical student. You're here to see if you can learn something about the crazy people. I can see that you're more anxious than I am. I don't think it's going to work then, is it?"

My skill might have been embryonic, but at many centers, psychoanalysts developed enormous skill in speaking with severely ill patients, including those with schizophrenia. We will discuss these skills in the next chapter. Many believed that medications that reduced the intensity of psychotic symptoms would diminish the internal conflict that makes psychodynamic psychotherapy possible. Patients who are indifferent to their symptoms might be more difficult to treat than those who recognize their own behavior and thinking as the sources of their anxiety. Trials comparing psychotherapy versus drug therapy were proposed and some were initiated, but the results, for a variety of reasons—patients too chronically ill, therapy too brief, or therapists too inexperienced—were considered inconclusive. Some centers therefore continued treatment wards that attempted to treat young patients without medications for several decades.

The Dramatic Results of Neuroleptic Medications

As a plethora of double-blind, placebo-controlled studies established their efficacy, the use of neuroleptics grew. The double-blind studies established that up to 70% of patients could be maintained out of the hospital in outpatient facilities while receiving neuroleptic drugs, compared to less than 20% of those who received placebo.[6] Neuroleptic drugs dramatically diminish the symptoms of schizophrenia and the effect is almost immediate, with the effect becoming maximal at about 6 weeks. The change has never been found to be any greater than Jean Delay and Pierre Deniker first described in 1952.[7] Patients do not lose their hallucinations and delusions, but their intensity and the amount of time spent thinking in that vein can decrease markedly. The impact on the lives of patients can be dramatic. Many are able to leave the hospital and resume at least partial employment. It was once hoped that patients might be able to stop the medications as they improved. That has not been the case. A small percentage have single episodes of psychosis from which they recover but such recoveries were well-known before the introduction of neuroleptic drugs. They do not appear to be a consequence of drug treatment. As patients returned to their families, partially treated, the families responded by demanding more services for them. The community mental health centers became a mainstay of their treatment, offering group and individual therapy along with drug treatment. Partial hospitals, boarding homes, and vocational assistance were added. In the United States, disability funding through Medicare and Medicaid were instituted. As mental hospitals became smaller, their bed availability decreased below the population's need and general hospitals took over the role of brief hospitalization during crises. Then in 1996 First Lady Rosalyn Carter and the National Alliance for the Mentally Ill began advocating for better treatment and, for the first time, for major support of biological research.

Therapeutic Effects Prompt Neuroscience Research

This social transformation was matched by scientific breakthroughs based on curiosity about the neuronal basis of the neuroleptic effect. It seemed that neuroscientists for the first time had a silver bullet, a drug that targeted psychosis, which they could use to identify which neurons were responsible for psychosis. The drugs could be given to laboratory animals, with the presumption that rodents would have the same neuronal effects as humans. Arvid Carlsson's discovery increased the recognition that psychoactive drugs might produce their effects through very specific reactions with the neurotransmitters and receptors of the brain's own circuitry and that a drug with a profound psychotropic effect, but with no known mechanism of action, could be used as a probe to discover the effects of a new neurotransmitter system. Ultimately, mechanisms of action for antidepressants, antianxiety drugs, opiates, stimulants, and cannabis would be found by this strategy. Paul Greengard shared the Nobel Prize with Carlsson and Eric Kandel, for showing that dopamine interacts with a specific class of dopamine receptors.

Most accounts of schizophrenia therefore emphasize the role of dopamine.[8] Although the complete description of the dopamine receptors took many decades to explicate, progress in the field was helped by the simultaneous interest of neuroscientists and neurologists in dopamine. Dopamine is an acronym for dihydroxyphenylacetic acid amine. A class of neurons synthesizes it for specific use as a neurotransmitter by adding a hydroxyl group to tyrosine, which is an essential amino acid. Essential means that you must eat the tyrosine; you cannot make it yourself from other chemicals in the body. It is difficult, however, to have a diet that is deficient in tyrosine, which is common in plant and animal-based proteins. Like acetylcholine, glutamate, and GABA, dopamine is stored in nerve terminals and then released onto the receptors of other neurons.

An entire class of neurotransmitters, called the catecholamines, is made from tyrosine. The class is best understood by considering that the neurons and cells that make catecholamines are different from most other nerve cells, which are part of a neural tube that forms early in development to become the spinal cord and brain. The cells destined to use catecholamines as their neurotransmitters form outside the tube, in an area called the neural crest. Some migrate into the brain and some migrate elsewhere into the body. Understanding that they are all close cousins, all of whose actions are affected by neuroleptic drugs, provides the rationale for the vast array of effects found in patients with schizophrenia who receive these drugs.

Antipsychotic Actions in the Brain

The ventral tegmental area innervates the temporal and frontal lobes, and its projections are thought to be involved in the principal antipsychotic actions of the neuroleptics. Dopamine is not a classic excitatory or inhibitory neurotransmitter, because it does not open or close ion channels directly. Rather it activates metabolic systems within the cells that use energy to exchange sodium and potassium. The net result is that the cells that receive a dopamine synapse become more responsive to other inputs. In small doses, this activity increases the ability of the person to respond to the environment. In children or adults who have attention-deficit/hyperactivity disorder (ADHD), as well as in normal persons who take stimulants, this effect improves performance. As the amount of dopamine increases, however, neurons can become bombarded by all the stimuli in the environment. The neuron is then less able to respond only to stimuli that are important. If inhibitory circuits are also deficient, then the probability of the kind of misjudgments that occur in psychosis is increased.

Dopamine cannot be measured directly in the living brain. Dopamine in the brain is metabolized to homovanillic acid, which eventually finds its way into the bloodstream where it can be measured. However, the measurement also reflects catecholamine activity outside the brain as well. Nonetheless, it provides a rough indication of the underlying dopaminergic neurotransmission in schizophrenia and in normal mental functioning. Homovanillic acid naturally increases when individuals are awake and alert, but also when they are under stress. It is part of the normal response of the brain when it needs to increase its sensitivity to stimuli. Catecholamines all over the body, including dopaminergic neurons of the ventral tegmental area, participate in the heightening of the body's responsiveness as part of its "fight or flight" response to danger.

Homovanillic acid levels of persons with schizophrenia range from high to low levels of normal, but they rarely exceed the upper range of normal. Higher levels are associated with increased occurrences of psychosis. Over longer periods of time higher levels are associated with more difficulty in maintaining independence in the community. A blockade of dopamine receptors by antipsychotic neuroleptic drugs results in improvement in sustained attention, as well as the decrease in the clinical symptoms of psychosis. Evoked potentials, including P50, become larger when antipsychotic neuroleptic drugs are administered to persons with schizophrenia. There is no change in the ratio of the test to conditioning amplitude, however. Thus, the mechanism does not involve the types of inhibitory and excitatory pathways we examined earlier in our investigation into the nature of inhibition in the hippocampus. There is actually little dopaminergic innervation of the hippocampus; the role of dopamine probably is centered in its innervation of the entorhinal cortex, the source of auditory information to the hippocampus. An increase in amplitude accompanied by a decrease in latency or time to the P50 peak from the occurrence of the stimulus would suggest that the drugs increased excitability of the entorhinal cortical neurons that project to the hippocampal neurons which generate P50. However, we observed increased latency, which suggests that excitability has been decreased. If neurons are hyperexcitable to stimuli, then they are discharging in response to many different stimuli, not only the auditory stimuli that we provide to generate P50. A neuron that has just responded to one stimulus cannot immediately respond to another stimulus, such as the click for P50. Therefore, the potential recorded at the cell surface diminishes in amplitude. The potential is said to be occluded by the other activity that the neuron has responded to. If excitability is diminished, the neuron is more likely to have been silent before the auditory stimulus arrives and therefore the P50 response is paradoxically larger. Persons with schizophrenia have significantly occluded P50 responses that are restored to normal levels when they are treated with neuroleptics. Ventral tegmental neurons form dendrite-to-dendrite synapses, in which they innervate each other and through mutual feed-back loops keep their firing rates quite low. This low rate of firing provides enough dopamine to keep other neurons sufficiently responsive to their inputs, but not enough to allow the system to go out of control. If the inputs to the ventral tegmental area become sufficiently strong, then there is a brief burst of activity in the ventral tegmental area that lasts until the self-inhibitory loops reassert themselves. Thus, in the best of circumstances, dopamine is only used in large amounts for emergencies, when the brain needs to register all stimuli, to try to find out as much as it can about unexpected or frightening changes in its surroundings.

The system can be circumvented by stimulant drugs. These drugs can release dopamine from synapses without the need for neurotransmission, which means that the feedback loops are no longer operative. Amphetamine was synthesized by German biochemists during World War II, to try to keep aircraft carrier pilots more alert. Amphetamine continues to be used for this purpose by the Air Force, because the pilots need to respond quickly and perform at high levels to fly military aircraft. Amphetamine not only releases dopamine, but it releases norepinephrine as well. Norepinephrine does innervate the hippocampus and, among other actions, it inhibits inhibitory interneurons. Thus, in addition to increased information flow, there is decreased inhibitory filtering. The amphetamine is self-administered by the pilots, which is problematic because it produces some feelings of euphoria, which the pilots then use to judge the dose. Unfortunately, there is great tolerance for the euphoric effect. In other words, ever-increasing doses are needed to repeat the feeling of euphoria. The pilots can then easily overdose themselves. The resultant flood of information leads to misjudgments, so that accidental bombings of friendly targets sometimes result, which are attributed to the use of amphetamine. Continued use of high-dose amphetamine leads to paranoid psychosis in most individuals, which, in addition to the anti-psychotic effects of the dopamine- blocking neuroleptic drugs, is used as evidence to support the role of dopamine in schizophrenia.

The blockade of dopamine receptors occurs to some extent at all five of the dopamine receptor subtypes, but the D2 receptor is the most sensi-tive. Chlorpromazine, the initial neuroleptic drug, was followed by an entire generation of drugs, over 20 of them, all of which were similarly effective. Their differences in potency, the amount needed to produce an effect, were directly related to their potency at D2 receptors. The ability to predict an effect as profound as the antipsychotic effect in schizo-phrenia based on effects at a single neurotransmitter receptor was a profound piece of evidence for a biological theory of schizophrenia.

Limitations of Antipsychotic Drugs

As with all medications, there were some limitations. First, postsynaptic blockade occurs immediately, but the full therapeutic effect takes about 6 to 8 weeks. During this period, plasma HVA levels gradually fall from the high normal levels that characterize people with acute schizophrenia to very low levels. Conversely, when patients are withdrawn from neuroleptic drugs, the antipsychotic effect persists for over 6 weeks, despite the fact that the medicine leaves the body in several days. The full antipsychotic effect therefore takes more than the postsynaptic blockade of the D2 receptor, but a substantial decrease in dopaminergic neurotransmission at all receptors. The remaining four receptor types are quite a bit less sensitive to antipsychotic drugs than D2 receptors. The mechanism by which neuroleptic drugs gradually decrease dopaminergic neurotransmission has been demonstrated in animal models. The dendrite autosynapses are blocked by antipsychotic drugs, just as other dopamine receptors are blocked. The result is that the ventral tegmental neurons increase their firing rate. That generates an increase in dopamine release, which increases the level of dopamine's brain metabolites, which is what Arvid Carlsson first measured and deduced to be the result of dopamine receptor blockade. Over the next several weeks, because of the continuing antipsychotic blockage of dopamine, the dopamine cells increase their excitability to a point where their membrane potential rises so high that they cannot be repolarized. They cannot then discharge and thus no more dopamine can be released.

The delay in onset of the full therapeutic effect could be viewed as a psychoeducational phenomenon. Perhaps it takes time for the patient to learn to take advantage of the effect of lower dopamine neurotransmis-sion. But the correlation with the rise and fall of HVA levels, and the similarity in the time course of effect between most individuals, suggests that it is primarily a biological phenomenon. Similarly, the time course of loss of effect when the drug is withdrawn is also mostly the same among individuals. The slow time course of the onset of effect is obviously problematic, but the partial effect with immediate administration of drugs because of postsynaptic blockade of D2 receptors is sufficient to help patients become well enough to leave fully supervised treatment facilities. Managed care insurance programs therefore have significantly shortened the treatment time for schizophrenia from a lifetime to 72 hours. There are several aspects to the time course of effect that have clinical significance. The first problem is the inexperienced psychiatrist who finds that a patient is doing well and suggests a reduction in neuroleptic drug. Interestingly enough, patients view a decrease or change in their medication as quite risky and are likely as not to resist the suggestion. If they do consent, they find they do fine with the reduced medication until their next appointment in 3 weeks. Three weeks without symptom return seems so promising that another reduction is proposed, until at about 6 weeks there is a return of psychosis. The return of symptoms is unexpected because the inexperienced psychiatrist does not understand the time course of the drug's effect.

There are also a small group of patients, about 20% in most health care systems, who do well on quite low doses of the dopamine-antagonist neuroleptic drugs. These patients take low doses and probably are receiving only enough to effect postsynaptic blockade. Because they do not have the longer time course of reversal of the presynaptic blockade to protect themselves when they miss a dose of medication, they are much more sensitive to lapses in taking the medication than patients with greater illness who are taking higher doses of drugs. Thus, the paradox is that patients with a very good prognosis, who seem to do well on low-dose medication, are also quite sensitive to problems when they miss a dose. Paul is one of those patients. He does quite well on low doses of risperidone, but if he misses a dose or two, he has problems.

Potential Side Effects

A major clinical problem is the side effects of the antidopaminergic neuroleptic drugs. We now return to the neuroembryology of the neural crest and all the other ways in which the brain and the body use catecholamine neurons (Figure 7-1). For example, dopamine is also involved in the regulation of movement; patients who lose the dopamine-producing cells of a brain area called the substantia nigra suffer from Parkinson disease, an illness characterized by slowed movements and tremors. Many persons with schizophrenia develop these same symptoms when they are treated with antipsychotic drugs. Another area of the brain that uses dopamine is the hypothalamus. The hypothalamus is connected to the pituitary by a network of special blood vessels that begins in the hypothalamus, as capillaries surrounding the nerve cells there, and end in the pituitary. Because this small circulation does not travel through the heart, it is called a portal circulation.

The hypothalamic neurons control the pituitary cells in a kind of primitive neurotransmission: they release dopamine into the portal circulation and it contacts dopamine receptors on the mammotrophe cells of the pituitary, the cells that release the hormone prolactin. Until pregnancy and lactation, the dopamine keeps the mammotrophes from secreting prolactin. Neuroleptics block the receptors, although not well because they are the less sensitive D1 type. Nevertheless, enough prolactin is released to stimulate a few drops of breast milk in some women. The first publication of the La Leche League, formed to help women return to breast-feeding, advocated chlorpromazine treatment as a tranquilizer to help women in hostile environments that discouraged breast-feeding, that is, the hospitals of the time. The recommendation has been dropped. While it may have partially worked by increasing prolactin, the neuroleptic crossed the breast into the milk and the infant ended up sedated, which decreased nursing, the best stimulus for producing mother's milk. You cannot get one dopamine effect without getting another one, generally a less desired one.

In addition to the dopamine neurons, the other catecholaminergic cousins become involved. Norepinephrine is one metabolic step past dopamine. The norepinephrine neurons of the locus coeruleus are also blocked by neuroleptics. Because norepinephrine blocks inhibition in the hippocampus, some of this anti-noradrenergic effect is helpful. However, norepinephrine also maintains mood and some of the depression that patients feel on neuroleptic drugs may be due to the blockade of this neurotransmitter. Another role of norepinephrine is in the sympathetic nervous system, which runs parallel to the spinal cord, just outside the vertebrae, and innervates blood vessels and other vital organs. Its effects are also antagonized by neuroleptic drugs, which can lead to low blood pressure, seen as dizziness when the patient stands up. A final set of more

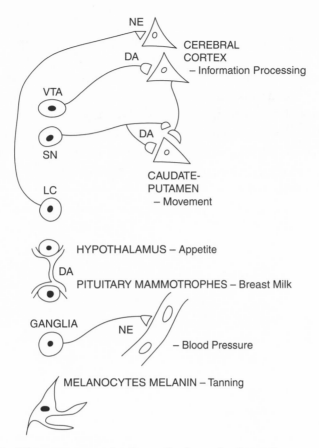

Figure 7-1. *The neurons and other cells that arise from the neural crest use catecholamines to perform various functions, all of which are impacted by antipsychotic drugs. The ventral tegmental area (VTA) neurons use dopamine (DA) to regulate information processing in the cerebral cortex. Blockade of dopamine here accounts for the antipsychotic effect. The substantia nigra (SN) provides dopamine to the caudate-putamen. Blockade of dopamine here produces the side effect of a movement disorder that resembles Parkinson disease. The locus coeruleus (LC) produces norepinephrine (NE), whose blockade by antipsychotic drugs results in decreased energy and loss of pleasure. In the hypothalamus, dopamine regulates appetite. Some dopamine is sent to the pituitary through small blood vessels, where it normally inhibits the mammotroph cells that make prolactin, a hormone that stimulates breast milk. Blockade of the dopamine by antipsychotic drugs can cause breast milk secretion. Norepinephrine is also made outside the brain in the sympathetic ganglia, where it regulates blood pressure. Finally, a polymer of catecholamines forms the skin pigment melanin. Antipsychotic drugs can inhibit melanocyte release of melanin, which results in sunburn. Thus, most of the effects of antipsychotic drugs reflect the common neuroembryology of this family of neurons.*

distant cousins is the melanocytes. These are the pigments containing cells of the skin, which polymerize catecholamines to make a pigment, melanin. Some pigment cells are in the substantia nigra (or black substance) and some are in the locus coeruleus (or blue place), both named because of their pigmented appearance in otherwise colorless living brain tissue. Neuroleptics block tanning, a problem until high-quality sunscreens were developed. Some neuroleptics can intercalate into the pigment polymer. This can cause skin discoloration or problems with vision, because of interference with retinal pigments. It is a reminder that chlorpromazine began its life as a purple dye.

8

Beyond the Dopamine Theory

The dopamine theory of schizophrenia grew out of the profound effects of the neuroleptic drugs, and it has had the predictive value of guiding the design of ever more potent drugs. Chlorpromazine required a mean daily dose of 400 to 800 mg. Haloperidol, the most potent of the D2 dopamine receptor antagonists, was equally as effective in doses of 1 to 5 mg. There have been many attempts to find definitive biological evidence that there is increase in dopamine transmission by some mechanism in schizophrenia. Increased dopamine metabolism, altered dopamine receptors, and genetic deficits in any molecule related to dopamine have been difficult to substantiate by any technique of molecular biology or brain imaging. This lack of evidence fits with the clinical observation that schizophrenia is not cured by these drugs.

In the absence of a biological model of schizophrenia that could lead beyond dopamine, the treatment of schizophrenia stayed unchanged for many decades. Psychiatric treatment mostly involved managing the side effects of the neuroleptics by being conservative with therapeutic doses. Movement disorder became the most problematic effect, because eventually about a third of patients developed a side effect also seen in Parkinson disease, a writhing involving the tongue, face, and sometimes the hands and limbs. The syndrome, called tardive dyskinesia, or late appearing abnormal movements, takes several years or decades to develop and is caused by chronic blockade of dopamine receptors in motor areas of the brain. Gradually, in response to the blockade, the neurons develop more neuroleptic receptors and become supersensitive to the dopamine that leaks through the blockade. Thus, removing the drug makes symptoms worse because then dopamine reaches all the receptors. Raising the dose of neuroleptic can temporarily obliterate the symptoms, but the supersensitivity gradually returns because the mechanism of sensitivity in response to receptor blockade remains.

A young woman with schizophrenia came to me because she was about to be married. Her mouth had started to pucker and she was afraid that she would have a visible dyskinesia when she marched down the aisle. If we took her off her medication, her dyskinesia would worsen and it would take many months to resolve. The dress has already been ordered! With her understanding, we increased her dose to make sure that she would not have dyskinesia, but then decreased it after the honeymoon.

Not all circumstances were as pleasant to deal with. For many, the disfigurement was not only cosmetic, but life threatening. The tongue has an interesting role in the body. It dances between the teeth, pushing food around them, and darting forward, dares to make t's and d's. Yet nearby are the mouth's sharpest incisors. No one fully understands how the tongue avoids an obvious fate. Yet when the teeth are gone, even in persons without schizophrenia, the tongue is no longer contained in the mouth. It begins writhing, searching movements. Dentures are helpful, but even with dentures this behavior increases. Tardive dyskinesia increases the behavior to the point where it can interfere with eating. The prevention is good dental care, including instruction of the dentist of the serious consequences of removing teeth in someone who has schizophrenia.

There was one neuroleptic that did not produce tardive dyskinesia: clozapine. It had been synthesized in Europe, where it was observed to produce less movement disorder, including dyskinesia, than chlorpromazine. In addition, it seemed to have a greater therapeutic effect, which was intriguing because the limitations of all other neuroleptics were now well known. It was not available for use in the United States, however, because it also caused the loss of white blood cells, which can result in death by infection. Led by two biological psychiatrists, John Kane and Herbert Meltzer, a landmark study in 1988 examined its effectiveness in schizophrenia in comparison to the other currently used neuroleptics.[1] Patients with a history of poor response to neuroleptics were treated with haloperidol to establish that they responded poorly. Then, the patients were treated either with chlorpromazine or clozapine. The test of a new medication against an effective older one is one of the most difficult for the new medication to pass, because there is already a considerable effect from the older medication. The fact that clozapine passed this test indicated that the biology of its effects needed to be investigated as vigorously as the anti-dopamine effects of the older neuroleptics.

The task has not been straightforward, despite the fact that more is known about neurotransmitter receptors than was known when chlorpromazine was first studied by Arvid Carlsson. Clozapine antagonizes most dopamine receptors, as well as norepinephrine receptors and many cholinergic and serotonergic receptors. There were two questions to resolve: Why was the movement disorder diminished, and why was the therapeutic effect increased? The answer to diminished movement disorder was proposed to be a decrease in the tightness of binding to the dopamine D2 receptor, and the increase in effect was proposed to be increased binding to serotonergic receptor, principally the 5HT2 receptor. Pharmaceutical companies jumped on the idea and a series of molecules meant to emulate these properties have formed a new generation of antipsychotic drugs: risperidone, ziprasidone, quetiapine, olanzapine, and aripiprazole. The first three most closely follow the diminished D2/enhanced 5HT2 formula. Olanzapine in addition tried to copy the overall structure of clozapine. Aripiprazole tried to capture the decreased D2 receptor binding motif by acting like dopamine at low doses (a property that pharmacologists call agonism) and blocking dopamine at high doses (called antagonism). The Food and Drug Administration does not require that new drugs surpass old ones, only that they have at least equal effect and no less safety. Clozapine was required to surpass chlorpromazine, because its safety was less than chlorpromazine's. None of these other new drugs surpassed older drugs in their initial tests, but all of them were safer than clozapine, in terms of their effects on white blood cells, and all of them produce less movement disorder than the older neuroleptics. A great deal of promotion accompanies new drugs and therefore there was some uncertainty as to whether the newer drugs, now called second-generation antipsychotics, truly had value over the older first-generation drugs. The National

Institute of Mental Health initiated the CATIE study to attempt to gather a large enough group of patients to test comparative efficacy and to assess comparative side effects.[2] Patients were accepted into the trial if they consented to be randomly assigned to at least two different treatments. There were no placebo controls and aripiprazole was not offered as a choice, because it was approved for use after the trial was well underway. Clozapine was not offered as a first choice, but it could be used later in the trial. A low dose of perphenazine, a first-generation drug, was offered as a first choice, but only to patients who did not have preexisting tardive dyskinesia. The other choices were the remaining second-generation drugs: risperidone, quetiapine, olanzapine, and ziprasidone.

The goal of the trial was to allow patients to stay with drugs that they and their psychiatrists agreed were effective and tolerable, but to move to second choices if the first choice was not effective. Third choices were also available. A principal measure of effectiveness was how long patients stayed with their first choice. Briefly, the first-generation drug perphenazine was as effective as the second-generation drugs, which were all equally effective, except for olanzapine, which appeared to be modestly more effective. At the second choice, clozapine was more effective than the other treatments. What we take from this study is that clozapine was the most effective and that olanzapine captured some of clozapine's increased efficacy.

The data from the study also suggested that movement disorder is only modestly greater with first-generation than second-generation drugs, provided that the first- generation drugs are used in relatively lower doses. When drugs like olanzapine and clozapine were not available, these drugs were used in quite high doses and produced excessive movement disorder, which was tolerated because some patients' psychoses could otherwise not be controlled. On the other hand, olanzapine and clozapine in particular produced high weight gain, approximately 20 pounds per year. Although the CATIE study did not continue long enough to establish the consequences of the weight gain, an increasing number of patients with consequences of what is now called the metabolic syndrome have appeared. The consequences included diabetes mellitus and coronary artery disease. Clozapine has also been associated with increased incidence of another heart disease, called myocarditis. And both clozapine and olanzapine can be quite sedating. In addition, clozapine requires biweekly blood samples to detect possible loss of white blood cells. As a result of all these problems, only about 10% of patients take clozapine at any given time, and the mechanism of its increased effect remains a mystery.

Clozapine has one other clinical outcome that is not shared with any other neuroleptic. Uniquely, a significant number of patients who take clozapine stop smoking.[3] The effect has been replicated in several studies and is more powerful than the effect of other antismoking treatment, including antidepressants, nicotinic skin patches, or chewing gum, in either the normal population or in patients with schizophrenia. The effect is a reminder that abuse of substances can reflect their specific interactions with the brain's own neurochemistry. Why do the patients stop smoking? Clozapine is not a nicotinic receptor agonist; it does not act like nicotine in any way. But it does increase the release of acetylcholine in the hippocampus, more effectively and at a relatively lower dose than any other neuroleptic. Only olanzapine approaches its efficacy. Clozapine is also the only neuroleptic that causes the suppression of the P50 response to normalize. The effect takes several weeks to months, but it often takes that long for the dose of clozapine to reach therapeutic levels. In animals, the effect can be observed immediately.

The mechanism of increased release of acetylcholine is not known, but one of the many actions of clozapine is to block serotonin 5HT3 receptors, as pointed out to me by my colleague Lawrence Adler. These receptors are located on the nerve terminals of many different kinds of neurons, including the nerve terminals of the cholinergic medial septal neurons that project to hippocampal interneurons. Blockade of the 5HT3 receptor increases the release of acetylcholine in the hippocampus, which may be the mechanism of clozapine's effect. Whether this effect in turn accounts for decreased smoking and increased antipsychotic effectiveness remains to be examined. Nicotine is not an effective drug for schizophrenia, because of its problem with desensitization. Thus, the substitution of acetylcholine for nicotine is a possible explanation for the improvement observed with clozapine in those patients who smoke. In patients who do not smoke, improvement would also be expected to occur with increased acetylcholine release. One study did find that patients who smoke are more likely to respond to clozapine.

Treatment Progress of Rachel and Paul

Rachel's treatment was by most measures successful. After the diagnosis was established, she was placed on a moderate dose of a first-generation drug. This treatment was sufficient to allow her to live independently without the need for any further hospitalizations. Nonetheless, she was not fully remitted. She could no longer work as a teacher, and she therefore receives social security disability payments. She had significant bradykinesia, a Parkinson-like side effect of her medication, which made her appear slow and awkward. Her personal hygiene was marginal. Although no particular symptom stood out, the overall impression was of someone with a mental illness. About a decade ago her treatment was changed to clozapine. She had a remarkable improvement in several aspects. First, her movements became more spontaneous and less awkward, and her face became more lively and expressive. Second, she lost much of the constriction in her thinking. She planned a trip to Europe to see a friend from college. Her personal hygiene became impeccable. Third, she resumed a creative role that she had experienced briefly in college, and she began to revise stories about herself that she had written in those days. The clozapine also helped in her resolve to stop smoking, which further improved her appearance. Rachel is easy to talk with. Her warmth is palpable, and I look forward to our sessions.

There were some side effects to reckon with. She gained 15 pounds, which she continues to battle with exercise. She also became troubled by obsessive-compulsive symptoms. She could not leave her house without returning to check several times whether she had locked the door. This symptom sometimes occurs with drugs that block neurotransmission by serotonin, and it responded to treatment with a serotonin reuptake inhibitor, which prevents serotonin from being transported back into the terminal of the neuron that just released it, thereby prolonging its effect.

Paul's treatment has had mixed success. He initially responded quite well to a low dose of risperidone, the range of dose associated only with postsynaptic blockade. Because of the low dose, he had no movement disorder and no other side effects. The thoughts of the snakes never left him, but his life moved on. He did not return to school, but he learned how to install sprinkler systems. With his mother's help, he started his own business by investing in his own truck. During the summer, he often hires a helper from a local family. Nevertheless, we have had to hospitalize him briefly every 2 to 3 years. If he misses one or two doses of risperidone, the snakes seize control of his mind. He becomes terrorized. He isolates himself in his apartment, and when his mother comes to extricate him, he becomes angry and resistive. Several times she has had to call the police to help bring him to the hospital. There, with reinstitution of his medication, he rapidly recovers and has little memory of what has happened. We have explored all other alternatives to low-dose risperidone, such as second-generation drugs and long-acting injectable preparations, but without success.

Beyond Dopamine

The story of clozapine is important because it is the first step toward discovery of antipsychotic drugs that move beyond the dopamine mechanism. The genetic information that we reviewed in a previous chapter has never been utilized to design new treatments for schizophrenia. Drugs directed to several aspects of clozapine's many actions are also being tested in early clinical studies. Because of the unique interaction between clozapine, smoking, and P50 inhibition, we decided to investigate whether some of its effects could be captured by direct activation of $\alpha 7$ receptors.

In Chapter 3, we used the analogy of a computer malfunction to understand the impact of sensory gating disturbance and deficient $\alpha 7$-nicotinic receptors on brain function in schizophrenia. Diagnosis of the problem chip is a first step, but it requires insertion of a new part to verify the location of the malfunction. An $\alpha 7$-nicotinic agonist, a drug that specifically activates $\alpha 7$-nicotonic receptors, would reveal to what extent activation of this receptor would normalize sensory gating and then reverse the other signs and symptoms of schizophrenia. Nicotine itself activates $\alpha 7$-nicotinic receptors, but because it was designed through evolution as a toxin it is not very effective or safe as a therapeutic drug.

I spent a great deal of time trying to talk pharmaceutical companies into making an $\alpha 7$-nicotinic agonist. Their ability to synthesize new molecules and to test their safety and effectiveness in animal models is unparalleled. They all listened to my seminars, but in the end refused. They explained that new therapeutic targets, regardless of their potential, are too risky for the multimillion dollar investment required for a new drug's development, when viewed relative to therapeutic possibilities of drugs for already evaluated targets, not only for schizophrenia but for all the other illnesses that can be treated with drugs. As a result, all of the current drugs for schizophrenia are dopamine D2 receptor antagonists and the enormous pharmaceutical industry investment in their development and marketing has not served the treatment of most people with schizophrenia beyond what two psychiatrists first observed with chlorpromazine in the 1950s.

But one non-dopamine-related compound has been developed at the University of Florida by Professor William Kem. Bill's first project as a graduate student was to investigate a small sea worm that lives in Puget Sound. He discovered that the worm poisoned other sea animals by injecting them with anabaseine, a compound similar to nicotine. Just as the tobacco plant had evolved the chemistry of nicotine to poison caterpillars, so had the worm evolved anabaseine as its weapon. Both nicotine and anabaseine inactivate nicotinic receptors in their prey's muscles, and both are examples of parallel evolution of the same mechanism in a plant and in an invertebrate. Ants also make anabaseine. Kem added other chemical groups to the anabaseine structure, which altered its properties just enough to make it more selective for $\alpha7$-receptors. Because it is less fat soluble, it causes less receptor inactivation than nicotine.

The final product, 3-(2,4 dimethoxybenzylidene)-anabaseine, DMXB-A, was the new ingredient we needed to test the nicotinic receptor deficiency hypothesis of sensory gating dysfunction in schizophrenia. But before any drug is tested in humans, its safety must be first tested in animals. The drug had been given to normal people in Wales, but before patients in the United States could receive it, the U.S. Food and Drug Administration (FDA) required animal testing in a U.S. laboratory—40 dogs and 80 rats. The pet industry breeds dogs, but many have scratches on their coat or a torn ear, and they cannot be sold as pets. These "seconds," as they would be called in the clothing industry, are sold for product testing, most of them for cosmetic testing. Fewer than 1 in 10 is used for medical research. The dogs were small beagles, chosen to conserve the expensive drug because it is given in doses determined by the animal's weight. Dr. James Stevens, our veterinarian, chose four young women, students at a laboratory animal care technician training program to care for the dogs. Each day every dog had to be held and a tablet of the drug placed in its mouth. Three weeks into the 4-week trial, Jim called. "The women want a grief therapist," he said. "They are beginning to think about what will happen to the dogs next week." At the end of 4 weeks, the dogs received an overdose of barbiturates. We were required to examine tissue from all of their organs under the microscope to detect any damage caused by the drug.

The private foundations named in the acknowledgments and the National Institute of Mental Health supported the cost of the trial, but there was no money for a grief therapist. I asked if I could do it. My psychiatric training has its occasional practical value. The women and I talked about their new identities as laboratory professionals, and we discussed how the first patients would be volunteering to take a drug that no one had taken before and whose safety could be judged only by their work with the dogs. The patients' willingness impressed them as courageous. Suddenly, one woman looked at me and said, "Let us show you the dogs."

Marshall Beagles weigh about 10 pounds fully grown and look like puppies. One dog could jump higher than the rest and seemed to be saying, "Play with me! Play with me!" "You haven't named the dogs have you?" I asked. "Well, just one," said the women pointing to the jumper: "He's 'Captain.'" Jim told the women that they did not need to help on the final day. The veterinarian technicians said they would do it, but the four young women resolved to stay with their dogs until the end. The tests on their tissues showed no damage, and the drug was approved for human study.

Paul and Rachel both agreed to participate in the first study, conducted by my colleague, Dr. Ann Olincy.[4] The initial trial was a proof of principle. The goal was to see if the drug had an effect consistent with our hypothesis of the consequences of α7-deficiency, rather than to initiate a new drug treatment for schizophrenia. Each patient came to our laboratory three times. On each day, their P50 responses were recorded, they took neurocognitive tests, and we rated their clinical systems. One day they received a placebo, another day a low dose of drug, and a third day a higher dose. Only the pharmacist knew the order of trials.

Dr. Steven Marder of UCLA, a consultant on the test, told us that it was important to talk with the patients, because how and what they felt might be more informative than the test results. That advice turned out to be correct for Rachel. She did so well on the cognitive tests on all 3 days that we could not see a drug effect, but she called me one evening after spending a day in our laboratory to tell me that the drug she had taken that day had helped her concentrate, and she was at that moment sitting down to work on some writing that she had not been able to concentrate on for many months. I told her that I was glad that she was having a good day, and that alone justified the drug trials, but for all I knew she might have taken a placebo. "It's not a placebo," she said. She felt that she could distinguish the effect from both clozapine and nicotine months later when we broke the code for the drug administration; it turned out that she had taken the higher dose that morning.

There is much that we do not know about the drug. We have learned that it normalizes the sensory gating deficit and that it improves cognitive function, particularly attention, and that the intensity of hallucinations decreases markedly, even for patients already on dopamine D2 receptor antagonist antipsychotic drugs.

We do not know if the drug will have long-term beneficial effects, as promising as the initial effects might be. However, we have minimally fulfilled the computer repairman's chip replacement tests, and the brain seems to work better. However, Rachel was by no means cured of her schizophrenia. Paul also took the drug, and he scored better on the cognitive tests, but he did not say that he felt better. Paul, like Rachel, went home to do some computer work that he had been neglecting, but he continued to mention that he was still concerned about his neighbor, whose children had the television playing too loudly.

There is a profound difference between the role of α7-nicotinic receptors in the brain and a malfunctioning chip. The chip can be easily replaced, even while the computer is running, but the α7-nicotinic receptor is not only involved in how the brain operates but also how it was formed during development. The developmental effects of a deficit in the receptor cannot be remedied by giving a drug to an adult patient. We will consider that aspect in a subsequent chapter.

9

Talking with a Person Who Has Schizophrenia

My son, Aaron, a student, was in nursing school and had a 1-week rotation on a psychiatry service. A man with schizophrenia had been admitted. He had been living in his automobile for 10 years and had not been treated during that time. On Monday he refused to talk to Aaron, which precipitated a call to me for advice. I told Aaron to bring a deck of cards the next day and no money. On Tuesday, they played gin rummy all afternoon. Aaron called to tell me what had happened and explained that he had to obtain the patient's history and fill out a questionnaire on his nursing care needs. Again I told Aaron to bring a deck of cards and no money, and the man would tell him his life story. Aaron called Wednesday night to tell me that, while they played cards, he had learned the man's life story and why he had come into the hospital. The police had to clean up the neighborhood because of the construction of new housing and had given him the choice between a hospital evaluation and jail. How can I get my questionnaire filled out, asked my son. Just bring a deck of cards, no money, and your questionnaire, was my advice. Thursday night's report was that they had played cards once again but this time filled out all the forms. Aaron told me that no other student had reached the level of interaction that he had achieved. What should I do on

Friday, he asked. Bring the cards, but make sure to leave your wallet at home, I said. Aaron called that night to tell me that the man wanted to play for money and became upset when Aaron told him that he had left his wallet at home. So he gave the man the cards, but he would not talk to Aaron anymore.

This story is instructive about how to talk with a person who has schizophrenia. The engagement is almost always a combination of reaching mutual comfort and exchanging practical information. Many persons with schizophrenia cannot process information well enough to form meaningful social interactions. They are perceived as distant, perhaps confused, easily angered, and negative. The negativity is a reluctance or sometimes a refusal to participate in new or unfamiliar activities. This negativism occurs despite the patient's self-proclaimed boredom and wish to have friends.

The person who wishes to interact with another person who has schizophrenia must learn to find a place of mutual comfort. For the patient this means the other person must be seen as practically helpful, but not intrusive. That prescription is no different from any human interaction for which mutual beneficence and mutual respect are key factors. What is different for an interaction with a person who has schizophrenia is the vulnerability of the person with schizophrenia and the corresponding fear of the other person. The patient easily lapses into negativism or paranoia when information-processing capabilities are overloaded. These lapses, often accompanied by anger, have the intended and also unintended effect of making the other person retreat.

Finding Safety for Rachel

As a condition of treating Rachel, who has three small children, I met with her and her mother several times to talk about ground rules. To be certain that Rachel and her children were safe, I had to be able to hear from her mother if she thought that Rachel was not doing well. It seemed reasonable enough, and for a year I did not hear from her mother. Rachel came to see me once or twice a week and complied well with her medication. We used the time productively. Persons with schizophrenia do not have many other people in their lives who are willing to speak with them without judgment and who have the patience, week after week, to hear paranoid complaints. For Rachel, it was her sister-in-law Sarah who could set off her rage. Sarah was always trying to be the center of the family, Sarah never acknowledged her, Sarah was always imitating her dress, her decorating, and her choice of friends. Sarah stayed in the foreground of our conversation for many months. What I was trying to do, however, was to enrich her view of her family beyond Sarah. Paranoia causes people to fixate all their mental energy on the target of their paranoia, to the exclusion of a broader view of what is available to them in their life. If you explode as her mother might—"Enough about Sarah!"—it does not diminish the intensity of the preoccupation. Instead, it is better to model a different view. Gradually, the whole family came into perspective. There were others in the family she could interact with, including her nephew, Sarah's son. Sarah's hold on her mind diminished and she was ready for an interpretation: "Perhaps Sarah is insecure," I said. "That's what Mother said," she replied, "but I didn't believe it until now." The work with her on Sarah was part of a larger plan to identify a role for Rachel, one that she would fulfill and give her life meaning. Sometimes the role is obvious. For Rachel, it was taking care of her three children. Her husband had divorced her as she became more ill, following the birth of her third daughter, and she had a major responsibility. Her family, including Sarah, was actually quite accepting and helpful to her. Her oldest son became self-reliant and could work directly with his grandmother as well as with Rachel.

Rachel had graduated from an exclusive liberal arts college and majored in writing. During the treatment, she brought me some of what she had written as an undergraduate. One story involved a girl who learned to perform cartwheels and handsprings in her effort to please her father. Her father was a warm, successful man, who prodded his children to emulate his success, often by teasing them. Although Rachel had never had to work because of the family's affluence, she had learned early that she needed to work hard to please her mother and father. The three children were one measure of what she had achieved and therefore our work often centered on raising them. Single parents have difficulty setting limits, because there is no one with whom they can confer to balance rigidity and warmth. Rachel learned to use me for guidance, a second example of the kind of practical help that is important for the person who has schizophrenia to gain from a therapeutic relationship.

Not all efforts were successful. Rachel bought chocolates from a local shop and became friendly with the owner so much so that the owner offered her a job one day. The shop featured over a 100 chocolates, with generally 4 to 5 of any variety. They were placed on shelves in groups, but the locations were not marked. Customers might ask for a specific one or for an explanation of differences between them. Prices were also not marked, but instead were simply known to the owner, who would tell them once or twice to the clerks and then expect them to know them as well. The clerks quickly learned this information, but for Rachel the cognitive load was overwhelming. She could comprehend and tell me about the magnitude of the task, but she could not master it. Cognitive difficulties of persons with schizophrenia include difficulty with short-term episodic memory tasks like learning the location and prices of the chocolates. The cognitive symptoms of schizophrenia are not particularly responsive to medication and there was little I could do to help her with the task. She recognized that the owner was giving her as much opportunity to succeed as possible, but in the end she recognized that she did not have the cognitive ability to learn the job well enough, and she resigned. People with schizophrenia like Rachel, who try every day to make what they can out of life, are the people with whom I value working.

During the treatment, her psychosis would wax and wane. It was generally worse when I was out of town, because the routine of coming once or twice per week to see me encouraged her to fill her prescriptions regularly and to make sure that she had medication and took it. When she would become stressed she would hear voices, sometimes derogatory and other times just filling her mind with repeated words, like "Happy Birthday." Such repeatings are quite common in persons with schizophrenia, particularly during periods of relative remission of their illness. Her medication was generally effective in treating this aspect of her illness, perhaps at the expense of some of her cognitive abilities. As we know from our discussion of dopamine, there is little evidence that dopamine is the major abnormal element in schizophrenia. If a person who did not have schizophrenia had gone to work in the chocolate shop, it is possible that the stress of learning the job would have led to increased dopamine levels, which would have helped that person be more vigilant and thus better able to remember which chocolate went where. I sometimes wonder if our neuroleptic medications, without which Rachel would have long ago been removed from her family, are nonetheless not the best treatment for schizophrenia. I think people will look back on the early twenty-first century incredulous that we took from persons with schizophrenia one of their normal coping mechanisms: dopamine! True, we have books like this one and its predecessors and learned journals that advocate dopamine blockade, but then George Washington's physicians, who bled him to death to try to save him, had their books, journals, and meetings to help them learn the latest rationale and technique for their treatments.

All of the second-generation drugs cause weight gain, because of their effects on hypothalamic centers that control appetite. In order to keep her weight normal, Rachel would exercise and diet, but as she aged, as for all of us, she had increasing difficulty keeping her weight under control. She therefore used the minimum amount of drug possible, which sometimes resulted in relapses. Her relapses were generally brief, lasting an hour or two until her son or mother could persuade her to take more medication. One of them lasted a bit longer and her mother called me, and I asked her to bring Rachel in to see me. The experience was humiliating for Rachel. She was angry with me and with her mother for talking about her. She accused me of taking her mother's side and of violating her confidentiality. Although she remembered that we had agreed at the beginning of treatment that her mother could call me if her mother felt that either Rachel or the children needed help, she was upset by what had happened.

There is no easy answer to the dilemma of how to handle safety in the psychotherapy of a person with any serious illness, but paranoia makes the problem all the trickier. Safety issues are paramount, but patients do best in treatment if they feel comfortable that what is said and done in therapy is under their control. In retrospect, it might have been better if I would have told Rachel's mother that the safety and well-being of Rachel and her children was something that I could not be involved in. Rachel's mother and her family would need to make other arrangements for that aspect of her care. I would be responsible only for making sure that she had good treatment in her relationship with me. Some treatment teams use what it called a therapist/administrator split. The therapist is responsible for the psychotherapeutic parts of the treatment, while the administrator handles safety, including the prescription of medication. For about a year after this incident when her mother brought her to see me, Rachel worked with a psychologist, while I continued to prescribe her medication and handle crises with her mother. In that position, I could be much more active with her family. On one occasion, Rachel brought one of her brothers in to see me, to learn how to adjust her medications during a brief relapse. It was another example of Rachel's ceaseless efforts to improve her life. She took advantage of the breakdown in our relationship to have me educate other family members to support her. She did not want her sometimes paranoid relationship with her mother to prevent her from getting help when she needed it.

All therapists encounter problems in the way they interact with patients, some of which stem from their own personal issues. For me, the problem is that I do not like people angry with me. I therefore work hard to make sure that my patients do not get angry with me. One of my patients pointed out that my skill in protecting myself deprived her of the opportunity to be angry and to learn about her anger. One of the learning experiences that therapists can gain from a patient like Rachel is that patients benefit from being angry. Rachel shouted at me one day that I had violated her confidence, that I was the tool of her family, and that she deserved a better psychiatrist, one that would be her psychiatrist and not her family's. I offered to find her one and she replied that she was perfectly capable of doing that herself and stormed out of my office. She called later that day and told me that she had thought about what she had said. She could not get over her mother's intrusion or my acceptance of it, but she could also see that I was genuinely interested in her and that our relationship was too important for her to discard. She returned to see me.

For psychiatrists who treat persons with schizophrenia, there are some requirements and some rewards. The requirements are patience, because problems are quite recurrent and, for many people, the continuing saga of the paranoid view of the world becomes boring. When patience fails, I rely on my neurobiological interests. The playing out of sensory gating disturbance and Rachel's interesting response to low doses of neuroleptics keep me endlessly fascinated. But the reward is that her own efforts, helped to whatever extent by me, have allowed her to live independently, with no more than 5 days of hospitalization in the last 15 years. She has raised three children, all of whom have gone to college, and maintained the support of her family. When I see her with her mother and sons,

I realize all that she has accomplished for herself, and this is what sustains me in my work with her.

Expanding Paul's World

With Paul, it is different. He actually benefited more from working with his mother than me. Paul rarely brings up issues spontaneously. My first thought was that his mind was so preoccupied with the snakes that he had little mental capacity left for any other interaction. I therefore increased his medication a number of times, but it had little effect on his spontaneity. However, he seemed more comfortable, and his mother reported fewer angry outbursts at her and at his sister. She sensed that he was growing bored with his job repairing lawn mower engines, and she began to talk with him about sprinkler systems. She arranged for him to apprentice himself to a landscaper in their area, who, like the repair shop owner, could appreciate his mechanical ability. Recognizing the liability that Paul's illness could mean for his employees' health insurance, he arranged to make him an independent contractor. Paul then did not have to negotiate directly with homeowners; rather, he is a subcontractor for landscapers, who can value his work and do not mind his lack of emotional spontaneity. As he became active, and with the increased medication, the snakes have retreated into the background. After frequent relapses due to stopping medications, as described in the last chapter, he developed a methodical approach to the medication, and he has not had a relapse for a number of years.

The prevalence of schizophrenia is less in many underdeveloped countries than it is in the developed world. The ability of a person early in the course of his illness to find a niche where he is uniquely suited, in part because of his illness, often is as important as any psychotherapeutic intervention. The medication helps most in making Paul reliable. Before he began taking it regularly, he occasionally would be too upset to go to work, and then there would be problems with customers whose engines were not ready on time. Filling a niche requires filling it reliably, and the medication brings reliability to his life.

Part of treating schizophrenia is trying to reverse the inevitable constriction of interest that the illness seems to bring. The world becomes smaller and smaller under the influence of the delusions, just as Paul's world initially shrunk to his dormitory room. I therefore spend the time with him trying to expand it a little. The initial attempts were with his coworkers and their roles. He came to expect me to ask about the other gardeners, who they were and what they were doing. Over the summer, the details began to grow about their names and their idiosyncrasies. One benefit was that their behavior became more predictable to Paul, so that the gardener who cursed when one of Paul's sprinkler lines went through some soil that he had just graded was no longer seen as threatening. Another benefit was that Paul discovered one of the part-time gardeners who shared his reticence, and they began to eat together. Eventually, Paul hired him to work for him during his busy season. The psychological scaffolding around him and his own innate temperament make him appear reliable and unflappable, a paradox for one who began his adulthood unpredictably psychotic. It appealed to the sister of one of the landscapers he worked for, and they married. He now has two stepchildren to whom he is quite devoted. He is able to interest himself in their development, including their school activities and their friends, which has drawn him further into the world.

With both of these individuals, the treatment has not involved interpreting the meaning of the psychotic material. Neither Rachel nor Paul has been particularly interested in talking about it, and both tend to see it as nuisance material, a spam of the mind. Nor has it been obvious to me that there is some symbolic meaning to the symptoms. Rachel had seen *Star Trek* but she was not a fanatic, and Paul knew that snakes hid under rocks near his house, but they never bothered him. A snake in the garden and influence from the heavens are as biblical as one could imagine, and they are common themes for delusions and hallucinations for people with schizophrenia. Their universality suggests that they do not come from specific unconscious conflicts for either Paul or Rachel, but they do suggest that these themes are common in many peoples' psyches. For both Paul and Rachel there was an unusual element to the fear that I have seen only in acute schizophrenia, the fear that your thoughts are being controlled or that your mind is being taken from you. I once received a letter from a person with schizophrenia who asked that I join his movement to post signs on our homes to tell aliens not to enter. He felt that this action would protect people from having their minds stolen—analogous to the biblical account of marking homes for sparing of death during the Passover.

Neither Paul nor Rachel has offered me much insight into this symptom, which is called thought withdrawal if it involves thinking, or passivity if it involves actions. If there is a normal correlate, perhaps we can look again to religious conversion. Sometimes people describe letting God or Jesus into their heart and letting Him control their lives. I have also thought about it as a computer analogy. If there is a virus using large amounts of processor time, it slows down the systems. But if you can remove the virus, the programs you access can run more slowly. Perhaps during times of intense psychotic activity, reverberating psychotic thoughts are draining much of the brain's capabilities. Patients then experience their own thoughts as running slower and thus conclude that part of their mind has been stolen and in a way it has been pre-occupied. However, the virus intrudes into their own thoughts as well and can cause self-destructive or even homicidal actions.

For Paul and Rachel, there is little reason to be overly involved in their hallucinations and delusions, and there is a suspicion on my part that if I do become interested in them, I will only stimulate more hallucinations and delusions, the inverse of purposely trying to stimulate Paul's interest in the people around him. However, there are some circumstances in which I try to become more involved with hallucinations or delusions and that is when I suspect the patient is capable of violence.

Assessing Violence

Robert is a 31-year-old man whom I have treated for 10 years. He has been arrested three times: for threatening a tire repairman, for vanda-lizing the mailbox in his apartment, and for vandalizing the car of one of his neighbors. Robert first became psychotic in college, with vandalism of his fraternity the presenting feature. He is quite bright, with a parti-cular interest in football that is obsessional, rather than communicative. If I try to talk about football with him, I am overwhelmed by statistics, derogatory comments about the coach, and no real sense of the camar-aderie that two people might share who live in the same town as the football team. What I have come to learn about his violence is that it arises out of the same type of obsessive thinking. He can brood for months about how his neighbor laughed at him, left smelly garbage around, failed to clean up his junk mail, or stood in front of his mailbox to read the mail. He will then laugh and say, "I know, I know, get over it! That's what my dad tells me to do. It doesn't mean anything." It goes on like this for some time and then one day I get a call from his apartment manager that he has "done it again."

Although the people around him are enlightened and eschew stigma against mental illness, they are also afraid of his propensity for violence. For a long time, there was a violent act about once every 18 months. Just about the time that everyone would forget about the last act, Robert would strike out again. I pointed out to him that these occasional lapses were just enough to maintain his neighbors' fear of him and in fact to stigmatize him. What helps him is that the building has a high turnover of tenants. The landlord values a tenant who does not leave, and those who fear him are generally gone for other reasons within a year.

His broodings have all the hallmarks of psychotic violence. He dwells on the slights of the others around him, he feels that the slights are perpetrated because he looks like a homosexual (he actually has no sexual life), and he makes elaborate plans for retribution. In his case, these always involve acts against property, not against the person, or we would have a more serious problem. Although the premeditation occurs over many months, the actual act is not planned. He becomes upset, generally at some perceived slight, and then acts suddenly and impulsively. However, the act takes full advantage of the months of rumination, and therefore it appears to have been planned to the last detail.

This pattern of activity was not stopped by treatment with conventional neuroleptics. However, it did respond to a second-generation neuroleptic, olanzapine, but it also probably diminished because of his age. He has now gone 5 years without a violent act, and he is able to work part time in a florist shop. We have learned to spend a great deal of time talking about his ruminations. Like most people contemplating violence, Robert dehumanizes his intended targets until they become caricatures that are easy to hate. We spend time talking about any targets to give them a human face. For example, he felt slighted because one neighbor was laughing when he got on the elevator. Who else was on the elevator? I asked. It turned out that the neighbor's wife and two small sons were on the elevator at the same time, and Robert came to realize that the family was laughing among themselves, not at him. Seeing the neighbor as the father of a small family made him a much less likely target for violence.

Theodore Kaczynski, the Unabomber, is an example of a psychotic person who committed significant violence, as did Cho Seung-Hui, the shooter at Virginia Polytechnic Institute. Both of them spent long periods of time in isolation, Kaczynski isolated in a Montana cabin and Seung-Hui estranged from his classmates in part because of his ethnic difference. Both of them saw psychiatrists for very brief periods of time as voluntary patients, but were not considered to be imminently dangerous. Neither of them continued with treatment. Most psychotic people, like Paul and Rachel, are not violent, and most violence is not committed by psychotic people, but rather by sociopaths, often under the influence of stimulants like methamphetamine. However, some persons with schizophrenia commit bizarre, intricately planned acts of violence. Because many such acts include suicide, we often do not know the diagnosis for certain. In Kaczynski's case, his suicide attempt in jail while he was awaiting trial was thwarted and therefore he had a diagnostic interview and the results were made public and led to commitment to a federal mental hospital. John Hinckley, who shot President Regan and two other federal officials, also received the diagnosis of schizophrenia in a subsequent trial. His isolation was more like Robert's. He was living at home and seeing a psychiatrist, but he managed to keep his violent plans secret from his family.

Despite the secrecy with which the plans are constructed, these individuals rarely keep their plans entirely hidden. They may deny all plans when asked directly, but they make sure that their plans are well broadcast in surprisingly public ways. Teachers of Eric Harris, the Columbine High School shooter, and Seung-Hui reported violent class compositions to school counselors. Harris and Dylan Klebold had a Web site. Kaczynski sent articles to the *New York Times* and the *Washington Post*. Hinckley wrote letters to Jody Foster, which she turned over to authorities.

The task for doctors and families is to detect the signs of the plan that leak out and then to work with patients to reduce violence. Like Robert, the patients will generally deny the importance of their violent fantasies and preoccupations when they are directly confronted about them. A better plan is to open the dialogue, so that the fantasy is played out as much as possible in words, rather than kept secretly for action. As the fantasy is revealed, the therapist can try to make the object of the violence as real a person as possible. As they prepared to march into Columbine High School, Harris saw a student whom he had gone to grade school with and told him to go home. The student understood the seriousness of the warning and tried to alert the police. The same student had seen his name on a targeted list on Harris's Web site a year earlier. When the police would not intervene then, he took it upon himself to get to know Harris and to establish a friendly relationship. That turned out to be a life-saving intervention for him.

This kind of intervention cannot be done in a single session, because it takes time for the violent fantasies to gradually leak out and then time to make the targets into real persons. There is also the unpredictable element of when the violence will occur. For Hinckley, it was an ultimatum from his parents about his habits. For Harris, it was being turned down by the Marine Corps because of an antidepressant in his urine test. These events trigger an increase in agitation, probably mediated by an increase in catecholamines, and then their violent plan breaks through into action.

Methamphetamine users, one of the most violent groups in our society, have an agitated psychosis because of their methamphetamine use, which increases dopamine and norepinephrine and also allows their violence to break through. The answer to violence is therefore prolonged treatment, with psychotherapy to detect and then discuss the full extent of the violent plans and with pharmacotherapy to prevent a chance event from causing a surge in catecholamines that leads to the breakthrough of violence. Most of the acts of violence at schools have come in the spring, as longer daylight increases catecholamines, a circadian rhythm regulated by the pineal gland.

The civil rights climate in the United States has discouraged mandatory treatment except for very brief periods of time for acutely violent patients. Psychiatry's equivocal record in the proper use of longer-term involuntary treatment is one of the reasons for this discouragement. A single violent act, without earlier indications, including earlier violent acts that come to the attention of police, is rare. Early violent acts, even if they seem to be trivial vandalism, should prompt the question of whether the individual has a developing mental illness. If so, mandated outpatient treatment, including an evaluation for medication and an extended psychotherapy, should be instituted. The treatment need not be coercive, but it should be extensive in terms of months and years, not days or weeks. The medications have many side effects, and therefore mandating them is problematic. However, as with Robert, when the patient has the goal of resuming a normal life or at least of leaving treatment, he comes to understand that avoidance of violent acts over the course of 12 to 24 months cannot occur without the aid of medication; with this realization comes compliance. Robert never forgets his medication now, because he knows it would mean the end of the job in the florist shop. Psychiatry needs to do a better job of outlining model treatment programs that judges can order for this purpose.[1] Currently, without such well-identified programs, judges are understandably reluctant to refer individuals who have committed relatively minor acts to long-term treatment. The effectiveness and cost of these programs could then be monitored as well, to make sure that they are effective.

Talking with persons with schizophrenia requires understanding the illness itself. As in Rachel's family, some members of the family are more sympathetic to the person who is ill than are others. Her brother Fred, who does not share the sensory gating deficit, is always particularly critical of her. For him, as for most critical family members, it is not what she does, but rather what she does not do. He can accept her positive symptoms, but he has great difficulty with her negative symptoms. If she would try as hard as he does, she could work, she could care for her children without using so much of their mother's energy, and she would not be so dependent on their father for money. Patients who had frequent relapses were studied in England and, paradoxically, patients who lived with families were found to be more likely to relapse than those who lived alone.[2] When the families were studied, this kind of critical attitude was found to distinguish them. A second paradox was that these families also spent more time together, over 20 hours per week, than families whose children had less relapse. These families were spending large amounts of time in one room, generally around the television, and had few outside interests. They responded well to multi-family psychoeducational groups, initially formed to teach the families about the negative as well as the positive symptoms of schizophrenia. They achieved socialization with each other within the groups, thus expanding their horizons as Paul's mother and I have tried to do individually with him.

The issue that is hardest to address in talking with a person who has schizophrenia comes up rarely, but when it does, it is important to tune into. For many patients there comes a time when they examine their life and the life that their siblings or friends from school achieved, and they wonder what has happened to them and why. A facile discussion of genes and neurotransmitters helps if the question is why did I lose touch with reality when my mother got angry with me, a question that Rachel might pose. It does not work when she compares her life to Susan's. Suicide occurs for many reasons in schizophrenia, but the prevalence is about 10% in the first 5 years of illness. Some patients respond to the voices telling them to kill themselves, an intrapsychic expression of their pain. Others, in a much more sobering moment, become discouraged with all that they have lost in their lives. For the therapist or family member, that is a difficult moment because often I fear that the patient is reading my mind, and that my discouragement has stimulated discouragement in them. Persons with schizophrenia have an uncanny sensitivity to small gestures of discouragement in others. There are times when my patience and interest are depleted, most often because of other circumstances in my life. If all is well, I get a call from Rachel the next day or from Paul's mother. Rachel wants to know if I am irritated with her. Paul's mother is similarly concerned. I wait until I feel I have my own personal reserves back, and then I call to tell her that I still have enthusiasm for her treatment, but I was worried about my research. Family members often construct impossibly ambitious schemes, sometimes at more effort and expense than they can bear, to try to rescue their child. I counsel them and myself that the person with this illness needs not a single heroic gesture, but a relationship titrated to last for many years.

10

Developmental Course of Schizophrenia

The treatments discussed up to this point, both those in current use and those in experimental investigation, have been directed at the neurobiology and psychology of schizophrenia in adulthood, when the illness most commonly appears. The results have transformed the lives of people like Rachel and Paul, but these effects lead to rehabilitation, rather than prevention or cure. Although everyone's life has limitless possibilities, including the lives of Rachel and Paul, there do seem to be aspects of their disability for which they can compensate, but never fully overcome. The abnormalities in the brains of people with schizophrenia, although subtle, are likely the result of developmental effects of genetic variants, including those in *CHRNA7*, that had many of their most profound effects when the nerve cells of the brain and their connections developed much earlier in life, long before the onset of illness.

One of the newer frontiers of science is the investigation of how the brain constructs itself. The brain, along with the rest of the body, begins as a single cell that contains enough information in its DNA not only to develop brain cells but also to make sure that they are properly connected with each other to begin their function at birth and to develop further over the next couple of decades. As difficult as it is to try to understand

165

how the brain works when it is fully developed, it is even more unfathom-able to understand how it grew from a single cell. The answer is not fully known, but it involves an interaction between the growth principles that work throughout the rest of the body by which one cell responds to hormones secreted by other cells, taking advantage of the unique capability of brain cells to influence each other's electrical activity. We shall again use the example of the cholingeric innervation of inhibitory interneurons of the hippocampus to illustrate these interactions, and how they go awry in schizophrenia.

After the sperm and egg combine to form the first cell of a new human being, the new cell, called the zygote, quickly begins to divide to form at first a small ball of cells. These cells, which are initially all the same, begin to change or differentiate to fulfill their specific role in the new human being. One group begins to take on the characteristics of future skin cells. Cell division and differentiation continue and from the future skin layer, called the ectoderm, the first future neurons, called neuroblasts, begin to develop. As they are leaving the ectodermal layer to begin to form a tube, called the neural tube, which will become the spinal cord and brain, they express the first α7-nicotinic receptors on their surface. The *CHRNA7* gene is present in the DNA of all cells, including the zygote, and could have been transcribed at any time into messenger RNA from the α7-nicotinic receptor protein. However, the selective turning on and turning off of genes is an important mechanism by which the future human being develops different kinds of cells at the correct time. The gene consists not only of the exons and introns that will be put together to make the messenger RNA but also a region of DNA just before the first exon called the promoter. The promoter is not transcribed into RNA, but rather it acts as a receptor for proteins that attach to it. This attachment is thought to twist the double-stranded DNA open just enough for the protein that transcribes the exons into messenger RNA to attach to one of the strands and begin its work of copying the DNA of the exons in messenger RNA (Figure 10-1). The *CHRNA7* promoter has a number of sites, each of them a particular sequence of the A, C, G, and T nucleotides that interact with different signal proteins. Many of these signal peptides are made only in nerve cells. Therefore, one of the ways that a cell begins acting like a brain cell, including making α7-nicotinic receptors, is that it makes signal peptides that are specific to the brain. One of the earliest signs of that occurrence is the expression of the α7-nicotinic receptor protein on its surface.

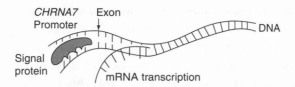

Figure 10-1. *Signal proteins control the transcription of DNA into messenger RNA (mRNA), the first step in the expression of a gene. The mRNA will make a specific protein, as coded in the DNA of the gene, that will guide cell function. The signal protein attaches to a specific spot in the promoter of the gene, because it fits the shape of a small portion of the genetic code there. The DNA then twists open to allow the exons of the gene, which contain the code for the protein, to be transcribed into mRNA.*

During development, expression of different signal proteins and receptors occurs not only in specific cells, but the expression is also turned on "just in time." Genes rarely act until they are needed, and genes that act out of sequence are often the cause of illness. Cancers, for example, involve the turning on of genes that were normally active during early development, but now are producing tissues that have no function. Cleft palate, on the other hand, is a developmental error that occurs when genes that direct tissues to reach the midline of the face are not turned on in time. The expression of α7-nicotinic receptors on future brain cells that occurs in the first few weeks of human development would seem to be an exception to this principle.[1] The axons that bring acetylcholine synapses to the brain cells that have α7-nicotinic receptors on their surface will not arrive until shortly before birth, over 8 months later. The receptors would seem to have been formed prematurely.

Clues from Unique Mice: The Dilute Brown Agouti

We can examine animals that have different numbers of α7-nicotinic receptors to see if these differences have any effect on the overall development of the brain. Because the most marked expression of α7-nicotinic receptors is on inhibitory interneurons of the hippocampus, they are a good index population to follow. In mice with the usual number of α7-nicotinic receptors, the interneurons are distributed throughout the cell layers of the CA3 region of the hippocampus and in apical dendrite and cellular region of CA1. One mouse strain, named for its coat, dilute brown agouti—a washed out brown fur with white tips—has only half the number of hippocampal α7-nicotinic receptors of other mice. In this mouse, there are few interneurons in CA3 and the interneurons in CA1 have migrated through the region and ended up at the very edge of the cell layer.[2] These changes are subtle and yet disturbing. This snapshot from adult life is mirrored by a more detailed look during pre- and post-birth developmental stages. The gestation of a mouse is only about 3 weeks, but the developmental expression of α7-nicotinic receptors begins a day later and is less robust in dilute brown agouti mice than in other mice.

This problem with α7-nicotinic receptor expression is linked to DNA polymorphisms in the mouse *CHRNA7* gene. Mice with two dilute brown agouti genes have about half the expression of *CHRNA7* as mice with the more normal version. If dilute brown agouti mice are bred to the more normal mice, their progeny have one dilute brown agouti *CHRNA7* and one normal *CHRNA7* and have about three-quarters of the expression of *CHRNA7* as normal mice.

Thus, we have the expression of α7-nicotinic receptors early during neuron migration and we know that α7-nicotinic receptor alterations are associated with alterations in neuron migration, but the piece that is missing is how the α7-nicotinic receptors are activated. Acetylcholine is not the only chemical that can activate α7-nicotinic receptors. Choline itself can do it, but only at quite high concentrations.[3] Choline levels are high in the amniotic fluid that bathes the fetus and in the fetus itself. These levels are high enough to activate α7-nicotinic receptors and there appears to be less desensitization, so that longer-lasting activations can be achieved than would occur if acetylcholine were activating the receptors. When choline or acetylcholine activates the receptor, the receptor molecules twist open to form a channel between them that allows calcium ions and other ions to enter the cell. The influx of these ions is needed for the cell to migrate. The same process using another nicotinic receptor, the α1-nicotinic receptor, admits calcium to muscle cells so that they can contract their muscle fibers.

But not only do the calcium ions help the neurons move, they also help them talk to each other. The neurons begin to form processes, their first exons and dendrites, that connect with each other to form synapses. Because they are future inhibitory interneurons, the inhibitory neurotransmitter GABA is used in their synapses. However, at this early stage in development, the nerve cells have a very high internal negative charge and therefore the GABA role is not inhibitory, but rather excitatory. The network between cells is just beginning to form and, as it does, activation of the nicotinic receptors activates the cells, and they release GABA onto their neighbors, which in turn are activated, and the network as a whole begins to become activated. A new brain has started to work. Even in adult life, neurons require activity to keep their role as neurons. Neurons that no longer receive stimulation, usually because the neurons that should be activating them have died, revert to ordinary cells, losing their processes and turning back into round cells.

In both mice and men, the nervous system will stay in this state of development throughout most of fetal life. Close to birth, another change occurs, also initiated by α7-nicotinic receptors. The heart of the hippocampus as a learning device is CA1, where the large pyramidal excitatory neurons are all lined up, perhaps the closest and straightest alignment of any cell layer in the brain. In late fetal life, the CA1 pyramidal neurons are covered with α7-nicotinic receptors. During this period of time, new receptors are forming on the cells, called glutamate receptors. These will become the excitatory receptors of the adult brain, and GABA receptors will become inhibitory. There are several different types of glutamate receptors, named for experimental drugs that specifically activate them, just as some acetylcholine receptors are called nicotinic, because nicotine can activate them.

The first type of glutamate receptor to be turned on is called NMDA, or N-methyl-D-aspartate, receptors. N-methyl-D-asparate is an experimental drug that activates this kind of glutamate receptor. NMDA receptors also admit calcium ions to the nerve cells and produce slow excitatory activations, just like the α7-nicotinic receptors. We now have synapses that contain both NMDA channels for calcium ions, which are activated by glutamate, and α7-nicotinic receptor channels for calcium ions, which are activated by choline. The α7-nicotinic activation is still required; it causes the development of a second class of glutamate receptor, kainate receptors, that admit only sodium ions to the cell. The α7-nicotinic receptors now disappear for the most part, the kainate receptors take over rapid signaling between neurons, and the NMDA receptors are activated only after intense stimulation of the kainate receptors, which means that the cell is receiving a lot of incoming information. At that point, activation of the NMDA receptors causes a long-lasting change in the cell's response, which many people feel is the neurobiological substrate of learning, as we discussed in the chapter on paranoia.

The dilute brown agouti mice do not have this expression of α7-nicotinic receptors on the pyramidal neurons of CA1. Consequently, they do not undergo the shift between a hippocampus that primarily has NMDA receptors to one that has kainate receptors. Dilute brown agouti mice are very slow learners, much slower than other mice, perhaps because of their failure to undergo this step in brain development.

Now, as the baby is about to be born, the nervous system is well enough developed to begin learning. The α7-receptors have done their job to help structure the nervous system. In fact, their expression during development is almost 10 times higher than it will be in adult life. Thus, to the extent that schizophrenia is caused by polymorphisms in the *CHRNA7*, the damage was likely done before the future patient was born.

However, there is still one last step for α7-nicotinic receptors during development. The cholinergic neurons from the medial septal nucleus, far below the hippocampus in the midbrain, are now reaching the interneurons. They are attracted to this region by a protein that the interneurons make called nerve growth factor (NGF). Their synapses, which release acetylcholine, also take up the NGF and send it back to the nucleus of the neuron. The signal becomes so important to the cholinergic neurons that, without it, they will die. If we block the continued activation of α7-nicotinic receptors, the interneurons respond by making more NGF and a related factor, brain-derived neurotrophic factor (BDNF). Thus, the hippocampal interneuron that has α7-nicotinic receptors and the medial septal nucleus that makes acetylcholine are now biologically interdependent on each other. Earlier in development, the α7-nicotinic receptor was critical for helping the inhibitory interneurons and principal excitatory neurons interact with each other. Now it is responsible for allowing older parts of the brain, the brainstem reticular formation and its extension to the midbrain, to talk to the hippocampus (Figure 10-2). These older parts of the brain serve to alert the hippocampus to what to pay attention, so that its unique ability to learn serves the most important needs of the new baby.

The hippocampus can be examined after death. Hippocampi from persons with schizophrenia show decreased α7-nicotinic receptor expression, as well as decreased expression of a number of neurochemicals associated with interneurons.[4] Some interneurons seem to be displaced into the white matter beneath the hippocampus and cerebral cortex, suggesting that they have not yet migrated into these areas, just as we

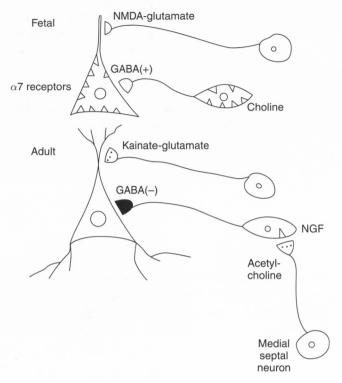

Figure 10-2. *During fetal life, α7-nicotinic receptors are widely expressed on both excitatory and inhibitory neurons. Their expression helps develop other synaptic pathways, including the transformation of GABA pathways from excitatory to inhibitory and the transformation of glutamatergic receptors from primarily NMDA type to kainate type. Because the cholinergic innervation has not yet formed, choline in the amniotic fluid is the activator of the α7-nicotinic receptors. During adult life, the expression of α7-nicotinic receptors is restricted to inhibitory neurons (as well as some presynaptic terminals that are not shown in the diagram). Activation of the receptors now comes from cholinergic fibers that originate in the medial septal nucleus. The α7 receptors are shown as small notches on the surface of the nerve cells.*

saw in the dilute brown agouti mice. Also, as we saw in these mice, the change from NMDA receptors to kainate glutamate receptors is not complete in the brains of persons who have schizophrenia.[5] It is staggering to believe that all this reflects what happened many years ago before the birth of the person who has now died, after a lifetime of mental illness. If we were attempting to prevent schizophrenia, it would seem that the fetal period would be the time to do it.

We can certainly think of things to do to make fetal brain development worse. The obvious intervention is nicotine itself, because it will very effectively desensitize the fetus's α7-nicotinic receptors. The transient activation that people who smoke receive from cigarettes depends on a sudden high dose. The fetus, partially protected by the placenta, receives a slow influx that primarily serves to inactivate receptors. In animal models, nicotine prevents the maturation of glutamate synapses, leaving them primarily as the NMDA type.[6] Human beings whose mothers smoked during their gestation show attentional and emotional difficulties that remain into adolescence.

First Efforts at Prevention

It is more challenging to think of interventions that would have positive effects. Certainly, we could intervene with specific α7-nicotinic receptor drugs, but drugs often have unintended side effects, and we would be particularly wary of anything that might even subtly disrupt the development of a human being. Choline is the substance that activates α7-nicotinic receptors during fetal development, and it is normally abundant in human bodies. It is part of the membranes of most cells, and it is found in abundance therefore in all meats, most dairy products, and in a number of other foods, including soybeans. It can be purchased in relatively pure form as a soy derivative in health food stores, and increasingly it is finding its way into multivitamins. The only time that human beings are thought to be deficient in choline is during pregnancy. The needs of the fetus for choline to build new cells are immense and women frequently cannot keep up with the demand. As cells are built, the levels of circulating choline, which is what activates α7-nicotinic receptors, can drop. This problem would be particularly problematic for the fetus that does not have an abundance of these receptors.

Our group therefore investigated whether choline supplementation would be helpful in the development of dilute brown agouti mice, as a test for whether it might be helpful for babies who had genetic risk for schizophrenia. The female mice were supplemented with double their usual dietary intake of choline from conception through weaning of their pups. The pups were then allowed to grow to adulthood on normal diets. Because dilute brown agouti mice have decreased numbers of α7-nicotinic receptors, they fail to inhibit the auditory response to paired sounds. However, dilute brown agouti mice who had received the supplemented diet during gestation and nursing inhibited the response to the second sound.

The effect could be viewed as analogous to the use of folic acid supplementation for the prevention of neural tube defects and cleft palate. These illnesses, like schizophrenia, are genetically based. While not all cases can be prevented, supplemental folic acid can cause the neural tube and the palate to close, despite the genetic defect. Mothers and fathers are not screened for the risk of transmitting these deficits, because some genetic causes might not be known and some could be genetic mutations that occur for the first time in that fetus. Men over 40 are more likely to father children with schizophrenia, because their sperm cells have gone through more cell divisions and hence have greater chance for a genetic error, because these cells divide constantly after puberty. Women make all their eggs before they are born, yet one more example of prudent planning ahead by females, and therefore their age is not as critical. Similarly, we would not screen mothers or fathers for the genetic risk of schizophrenia, but rather we would devise a treatment that is safe for all and effective for those who need it.

Choline supplementation during pregnancy is already widely touted on the Internet, not because of schizophrenia, but because of preliminary evidence of better learning and memory functions in children who receive it.[7] The Food and Drug Administration is prevented by Congress from regulating the advertising and sale of natural products, as long as they are not advocated for prevention or treatment of disease. Because we wished to study whether choline would decrease the risk of schizophrenia, we have obtained FDA approval to study the treatment as an experimental treatment. One of the problems is that schizophrenia takes up to 30 years to manifest, and it occurs in less than 1% of the population. We expect to be treating a lot of babies and waiting a long time before we know the answer.

Many Genes Are Involved

We mentioned in the chapter on genetics that there were many other genes associated with schizophrenia, not just *CHRNA7*. We have chosen it only as an example of how to think about schizophrenia as a neuro-biological illness. Although *CHRNA7* is the only candidate gene for schizophrenia that acts as a neurotransmitter receptor, most of the other genes are directly involved in the growth and development of the brain. One example is neuregulin1, *NRG1*, which is located on chromosome 8. Neuregulin was discovered because it seemed to be needed for the assembly of nicotinic receptors, but it has a broader role in the assembly of glutamate receptors as well. In postmortem samples of hippocampus, decreased neuregulin is correlated with a decreased number of α7-nicotinic receptors. Another gene—*DISC1* (Disrupted in Schizophrenia 1), was discovered in a microscopic or cytogenetic investigation of schizophrenia. Sometimes during recombination, instead of the two paired chromosomes exchanging arms, the exchange is made with an entirely different chromosome, which is called a balanced translocation. For example, there is a balanced translocation involving the *CHRNA7* region of chromosome 15 and chromosome 18 in an Italian family that gave rise to schizophrenia in a family in which this illness did not previously exist. For *DISC1*, the translocation involved chromosome 1 and 11 and resulted in the transmission of schizophrenia in family members who had this translocation. The presumption is that the sequence of one of the genes at the site of the translocation is disrupted. *DISC1* was a previously unknown gene, but it interacts with *NUDEL*, a gene known to be involved in neuronal migration. As we read in the chapter on genetics, a similar deletion during recombination can affect *CHRNA7*.

G72 on chromosome 13 was also a previously unknown gene, but its protein binds to D-amino acid oxidase, which regulates the levels of D-serine, which in turns regulates the activation of NMDA glutamate receptors. And close to *DISC1* on chromosome 1, but closer to the site where other investigations have shown evidence for linkage, is *RGS4*, Regulator of G-Protein Signaling 4. G-protein translates external hormone signaling, like activation of the α7-nicotinic receptor, but many other hormones and neurotransmitters as well, into signals that activate specific proteins to change cell functioning. It would be wonderful to say that all these genes interact to affect neuronal development in a consistent way that explains the pathology of schizophrenia, but that has not yet been established. Most of the genes, including *CHRNA7*, are part of the risk not only for schizophrenia, but for bipolar mood disorder as well. These two illnesses have significant overlapping symptoms, with many bipolar patients showing signs of psychosis and many patients with schizophrenia showing signs of the mood swings of bipolar disorder.

Another unresolved issue has been our inability to find the specific DNA changes that actually cause any of these genes to alter its function in schizophrenia. For *CHRNA7* we have found polymorphisms that alter function of the promoter region, but other groups have found that the valence of these polymorphisms is reversed. We find that they increase risk for illness, whereas others, working in different ethnic groups, find that they are protective. That situation occurs when you are very close to the DNA changes that convey illness but have not reached them yet, as we saw in Rachel's family in Chapter 5. Then nearby markers will show association with illness, but not always in the same direction. Since this problem has happened with each of these genes and in many other common genetic illnesses as well, some theoreticians have proposed that certain genes are commonly responsible for particular illnesses, but the actual changes in these genes might be different in various families. In Marfan syndrome, for example, while all the mutations are in *FNB1*, over 100 different mutations have been found, many of them in only one or two families.

The Developmental Course

We now have a baby born carrying the risk for schizophrenia. What does such a baby look like? Thanks to the ubiquitous use of home movies, there are now many motion pictures of trips home from the hospital of babies who 25 years later will turn out to have schizophrenia and, of course, many more movies of babies who will not have schizophrenia. The babies who will develop schizophrenia are floppier and less active than the babies who will not. These are fairly nonspecific changes and certainly not diagnostic of schizophrenia. Rather, they tell us that the brain is indeed already affected, but all we can see in terms of behavior is what newborns are capable of doing, moving around just a little bit and showing the beginnings of muscle tone.

The development of schizophrenia will have this characteristic throughout the life cycle. The illness appears in the context of the individual's developmental stage. As the individual develops, the symptoms of schizophrenia will become more manifest, with the full syndrome not appearing until early adulthood. What is not clear is whether all of the pathology is present at birth and then just revealed during development, or whether there are other critical milestones of development where further intervention is possible. The development is particularly hard on families, because they are often able to recognize that something is wrong and often seek help. They are usually told by well-intentioned pediatricians and school psychologists and psychiatrists as well that there is a wide range of development and that many normal children show these characteristics.

At each developmental step, however, the child falls further away from normal. The floppy infant becomes by the age of 6 a somewhat shy, but aggressive child, who is recognized as abnormal by the classroom teacher. There are learning difficulties and the pediatrician begins treatment with stimulants for attention-deficit/hyperactivity disorder (ADHD), particularly for the boys. By age 12 there are few friends, sometimes at best kindred spirits who have similar social problems. The girls are doing somewhat better, but by late childhood both boys and girls have more difficulty with anger than their siblings. Some of the girls are unusually aggressive. Boys with weapons are fairly common, but girls interested in weapons or threatening with kitchen knives are fairly rare in the general population.

Children are generally protected against psychosis. For example, ketamine is an anesthetic that causes psychosis in many adults, because it activates the sigma opiate receptor, releases dopamine and norepinephrine, and blocks NMDA receptors. It is similar to phencyclidine, also originally synthesized as an anesthetic, that is now banned because of the high frequency of psychotic reactions. Children under 12 years are much less likely to become psychotic than those over 12 and are often administered ketamine, because it is otherwise a safer anesthetic than most for this age group.

However, the protection is not absolute, and there are children who start hallucinating as the first sign of schizophrenia as early as 4 years of age. One youngster told my colleague Randy Ross to put his ear to the boy's head "to hear all the different voices inside of me." The illness in these children was not thought to be related to schizophrenia, because of its rareness and because most persons develop schizophrenia in later adolescence or early adulthood. However, there are strong family histories of schizophrenia in these children, often biparental. The early expression of schizophrenia in children with apparently higher genetic loading, despite the relative protection of children against psychosis, is typical of the effects of increased genetic loading on the onset of disease for most illnesses. Children also may lose the signs of schizophrenia, particularly after treatment, but early in the course of treatment in adolescents and adults there may also be a remission, which is most often temporary. Generally, children with earlier onset remain sicker all their lives.

By teenage years, the child is often depressed, socially withdrawn, and obsessional. The obsessionalism is seen as preoccupation with harmful events, which the child may try to forestall with various rituals, from reading the Bible to hand washing or avoidance of foods. The depression and obsessionalism often lead to treatment with antidepressants, as they are effective for these symptoms in adults. Treatment with stimulants for ADHD continues as well. Parents are increasingly bewildered. The child is on several drugs, there have been a number of family meetings, and the reassurance that he or she will grow out of it now seems hollow. Occasionally, they stop all medications and things look better. The stimulant, although helpful for the learning problems, may be making the child more agitated and even provoking some hallucinations. The antidepressant can also cause agitation. The probability of such a child, even with a family history of schizophrenia, having chronic schizophrenia is still low, perhaps 20%.

Then, there is an event that leads to the breakthrough of psychotic symptoms. It may not be as dramatic as the crystallization of paranoia that Harry Stack Sullivan feared. It is more often something that happens over the course of a year. Often there is a move or a separation, so that the individual loses contacts with the family and friends and community that sustained him or her. That is not unusual, as most young people make such moves for military service, education, or jobs. However, for the person who is developing schizophrenia, there is a change to a more overt psychosis. Here is where we entered Paul's life. A move back home may reverse the symptoms temporarily, but they generally return within a year.

The themes of development from child to adolescent to young adult run through the development of the illness as well, but they do not explain the significance of the various stations along the way. As the side effects of neuroleptic drugs began to diminish with the introduction of risperidone, it was hoped that their early administration might prevent the final development in psychosis. Much has been made of the risk–benefit of this intervention. First, the children are labeled preschizophrenic and, second, they are prescribed a drug with considerable side effects, when the probability of developing the chronic form of the illness is only about one in five. Furthermore, the current evidence suggests that at best the psychosis is delayed; it certainly is not prevented.

Another approach, now being used experimentally in several countries, could be called "getting to know you." The two programs, one in Norway and one in Australia, use massive public outreach campaigns to alert teachers, families, and classmates, to the early signs of schizophrenia.[8] Identified individuals come in for early counseling sessions. The supposition is that the duration of untreated psychosis is either neurobiologically or psychologically damaging and that early liaison with treatment facilities will lead to more timely treatment when illness takes hold. The Norwegian group has reported decreased suicide rates in young people in counties that have adopted this program. The program might also be expanded to consider early connection to children with violent fantasies. A system that provides universal, high-quality health care is obviously a prerequisite for such a program.

Between birth and adulthood there are no other obvious interventions for children who may later develop schizophrenia. What might be helpful seems obvious but has public health importance. Many families report head injuries or brain illnesses in their children who later develop schizophrenia. While head injuries are common in childhood, their repercussions are serious. The injuries range from automobile accidents to meningitis. Vaccinations against the more common causes of severe meningitis, such as hemophilus influenza and meningococcus, are good preventive measures, as are seatbelts and bicycle helmets. Substance abuse is also a possible predisposing factor, although an increase in the incidence of schizophrenia has not occurred with the increase in substance abuse in the United States. Nor has the common use of stimulants for ADHD increased the incidence, although such drugs can stimulate psychoses in vulnerable individuals. Nonetheless, there are important neurobiological changes ongoing during adolescence that appear to be different in children with schizophrenia. For example, there is a loss of neurons all over the cerebral cortex during adolescence that appears to be accelerated in children with schizophrenia. What causes this loss and whether there is an intervention that could stop it is unknown.

As individuals pass the age of 30, the incidence of schizophrenia falls dramatically. For men, it occurs only rarely. For women, there is some continuing postpartum psychosis, some of which is the first onset of schizophrenia. Women have a second small peak of incidence between ages 35 and 40, unrelated to pregnancy. These women are often thought to have depression, but the persistence of delusions and sometimes hallucinations is more typical of schizophrenia. Finally, in old age, the loss of hearing stimulates one final round of illness.

A 92-year-old man had been argumentative, but kind and generous throughout his life. He had run several businesses, developed lifelong friends, and acted as the head of his extended family until the death of his wife at the age of 89, and he then lived alone, but was in contact with the rest of the family. There was a family history of schizophrenia in a niece. Since his late 80s, and with time, he had increasing hearing loss. He began to become increasingly irritable with his sons. In his new apartment, he heard sounds of torture in the basement that he could not get out of his head. He cried when he described them. He had no signs of cortical atrophy or memory loss that would have suggested Alzheimer disease. I treated him with a neuroleptic, which diminished the voices, but it caused him to lose his balance and break his hip. He was considered too weak to undergo surgery and he spent the last year of his life in a nursing home, in the room next to a woman who was constantly screaming. He had known her as a younger man, and he had disliked her even then. He was my grandfather.

11

A Final Piece of Neurobiology—and a Final Thought

The aim of this book is to provide an introduction to biological research on schizophrenia, to see how it informs us about the experience of having schizophrenia and more broadly to see how it informs us about how our brains work. We understand now that schizophrenia is indeed a collection of small biological changes, any one of which might not be disastrous but whose combination leaves open the possibility of psychosis. When that possibility opens, it causes a change in one's view of the world that is not easily challenged, either by the person who has the illness or by others who wish to help.

I often consider how vulnerable all of us are to similar aberrations in our thinking. Any theory we make about our world is subject to errors in perception, like the sensory gating disturbance of schizophrenia, and to misconstrued convictions, including our own paranoia. But reality also steers us back from this abyss, you might insist. Persons with schizophrenia can steer themselves back also, often in emergencies when their help is needed most, but when their help is not urgently needed, they quickly lapse back into their delusions and hallucinations. Is it difficult to walk away from a serious conversation with someone who has schizo-phrenia and not wonder about the possibility of your own insanity.

There is no neurobiological bulwark that stands between us and this fate. Those that might exist, a robust inhibitory pathway or a well-integrated dopaminergic system, do not protect all of us and seem to be lacking in those of us who are the most troubled. Paul Meehl's formulation of a schizotaxia gene that would produce schizotypy or schizophrenia has been supported by a more complex genetics. The genetics tell us that most of us have at least one factor that has been associated in more than one study with the risk for schizophrenia.

People with schizophrenia who know that they have these uncertainties live with great dignity, and often with humor, between the times of terror. Their courage is what makes them most attractive to work with. For those of us without the diagnosis, the principles of their therapy may be helpful. First, do not take the future of your sanity for granted. The gods can test any or all of us at any time. Second, you can profit from a second look at what you perceive and a reconsideration of your most strongly held principles. Third, what is wild and crazy in your thoughts represents a mixture of ideas and reality that may be of immense value. There are few new ideas in our world and those who have the ability to hold several of them in their hippocampus for even a few seconds can end up seeing things in a more remarkable way. For the preservation of these capabilities among us, our species has transmitted several genetic variants through the last 1,000 generations. Persons who have schizophrenia, 1 in 100 of us, have paid a heavy price for these variants and the risk they entail. It is therefore incumbent upon the rest of us to use these abilities as wisely as we can.

Our fascination with persons who have schizophrenia is not simply that our thoughts, rational or irrational, use the same neuronal machinery or reflect the same human anxieties as theirs. The suspicion that the world as we know it is the creation of our own minds dissolves the comfortable assumption of a boundary between delusions and reality. Like Bishop Berkeley, we cannot resolve our dilemma, because any rational test is subject to the same existential uncertainty as our doubt. We must live with the anxiety that a harder reality may intrude suddenly and perhaps violently to dispel the autistic illusion that we have until now misnamed reality. Freud and Sullivan recognized the power that a paranoid delusion, like a religious conversion, holds over anxiety as a psychosis deepens. Just as we cannot test our reality rationally, we cannot dismiss the beliefs of profoundly psychotic persons as deluded. Their absolute conviction then paradoxically elicits our envy, because they may have truly seen the God that we can only imagine.

A Last Lesson from Neurobiology

For me, the variants in *CHRNA7* and the expression of the α7-nicotinic receptor have a special place that is the focus of this book. There is perhaps a sign that this primitive old mechanism that we study in rats has a special place in human life today. In the primate brain there is an immense development of the neocortex that is found in earlier small mammals, the precursors of our modern rodents. Just as reptiles, birds, and amphibians like frogs are mainly brainstem animals, so the rodent is primarily a hippocampal animal. For human beings, the cerebral cortex, with dozens of sulci (valleys) and gyri (hills), is an area for critical sorting of signals. A human being without a hippocampus cannot learn about the present, but a person without frontal neocortex loses judgment and the ability to forecast the consequences of his or her acts. The person without temporal neocortex has different, but equally significant defects, and is given over to all passions (feeding, fighting, fornication). The person who loses parietal neocortex loses the ability to understand intricacy. Occipital neocortex lesions preserve the ability to see, but the individual loses the ability to understand the significance of what he or she sees.

The neocortex clearly contains what it means to think as a human being. But like any great computer it requires a central processor that matches its capabilities. The processor for the neocortex is the thalamus, where all sensory information must pass before it comes to the primary sensory parts of the neocortex, which first analyze sight, sounds, and touch. The thalamus also collects information from the motor part of the cortex, which it sends to the spinal cord to perform the fine movements of the fingers. To other areas of the brain, such as the frontal cortex, it sends major connections as well. There is a single layer of inhibitory nerve cells that forms a sheath around the thalamus.[1] The dendrites of this nucleus intertwine, as do the dendrites of the reticular formation of the brain stem, and therefore it is called the reticular nucleus of the thalamus, although it is more a sheath than a nucleus. Axons leaving the thalamus below it send a small branch to these neurons and they in turn send their inhibitory axons back to the thalamus.

They are thus another example of a feedback inhibitory loop. The basic architecture of the nucleus does not change between rodents and humans. What changes is its expression of the α7-nicotinic receptor, which is minimal if at all present in rodents and which becomes robust in primates. In humans, the expression of α7-nicotinic receptors in the hippocampus is almost identical to that in rodents, but the expression in the thalamic reticular nucleus surpasses it and becomes the most marked site of expression of this receptor in the brain, and one that is decreased in schizophrenia.[2]

One could argue quite rightly that the hippocampal model that we developed earlier in this book is a very crude one for humans, who use the cerebral neocortex not the hippocampal archiocortex for most of their mental functions. The neocortex is a five-layered structure with two major levels of pyramidal neurons and many different types of inhibitory neurons. Neuronal processes frequently overlap several areas, increasing their interconnections. Its advantage over the hippocampus, which has three single layers that are separate from each other, must be enormous for complex information processing. Yet the oldest of the ligand-gated ion channel receptors and the most primitive of neurotransmitters are brought back to attend to the activation of these inhibitory neurons—and the expression is diminished in schizophrenia.

For me, this last twist of neurobiology suggests that it is still quite important for human beings to regulate the flow of information in their brains and that the cholinergic stimulation of inhibitory interneurons remains their major tool. Therefore, these simple sensory phenomena that we have examined in this book are very much part of how we use our brains and what it means to have a human brain, and thus to be a human being. As you already know, the subtitle of this book, *Schizophrenia as a Neuronal Process*, was based on the title of Sullivan's book, *Schizophrenia as a Human Process*. There is always a caution that when we get involved in biology we may lose the essence of humanity. After all, humans are more than a sum of their reflexes and feedback loops. Yet when we look carefully at a human brain, one of the changes we find over rodents is that we have enhanced the role of inhibition. It is therefore not surprising that its genetically determined variants have a significant role in human behavior.

It might seem odd to end our story with yet one more piece of neurobiology. We began the story from a philosophical and epistemological perspective on schizophrenia, and now we seem to end with one last detail about the way that nicotinic receptors work. However, the detail has a profound evolutionary significance. At least on this planet, the growth of our species' ability to think is unprecedented. With this growth we seem to have acquired an incidence of severe behavioral disorder that is quite high, in comparison with most other species, for whom suicide and killing of each other, outside of competitive male behavior during mating, are rare. If evolution were selecting for a better brain, then we might suppose that it would select for one more protected against behavioral disorder, rather than one more susceptible. Instead, evolution seems to have selected attributes that support enormous capacity, both to store information and to weave it into stories that organize the information, predict its future, and create new stories that have not been heard or seen before. Yet this enormous capacity is surprisingly unstable, easily overwhelmed by excess internal and external information. The sensory gating mechanisms that protected the hippo-campus of a more primitive rodent brain would need to be expanded quickly to accommodate the fast enlarging cerebral cortex of the primates that would become *Homo sapiens*. Evolution therefore brought forward a very primitive system, an ancient ligand-gated ion channel with the most ancient of all neurotransmitters to help the thalamus control the neocortex. It seems like a desperate, jerry-rigged solution. If we can process information in a much more sophisticated way than a rat, why do we use a variant of its sensory gating mechanism for our far more advanced cerebral cortex?

In fact, we have learned that many people can do without a sensory gating mechanism, or at least they can tolerate it being partly diminished by a dysfunctional *CHNRA7* gene on one chromosome. The conse-quences of such a deficiency are not altogether clear. For some, it appears to be psychosis, but for others it seems to be boundless curiosity and creativity, and for a few individuals it appears to be both. Perhaps it is not a coincidence that Albert Einstein had a mentally ill son and Søren Kierkegaard had a mentally ill mother. Evolution has left us with a range of capacities, seemingly based on the random assortment of alleles when eggs and sperm are made. We are frail in many ways. We begin life as a single cell, we are born defenseless, and we live with a brain that can easily become psychotic. These vulnerabilities are not restricted to a few unfortunate individuals. They are part of all of us.

Notes

Preface

1. P. S. Churchland, *Neurophilosophy: Toward a Unified Science of the Mind-Brain* (Cambridge, MA: MIT Press, 1989).

Chapter 1

1. Jewish Publication Society, *Tanakh—The Holy Scriptures* (Philadelphia: The Jewish Publication Society, 1985).
2. *The Trial of Jeanne d'Arc*, translated into English from the original Latin and French documents by W. P. Barrett (New York: Gothman House, 1932), 51; http://www.fordham.edu/halsall/basis/joanofarc-trial.html.
3. Eugen Bleuler, *Dementia Praecox oder Gruppe der Schizophrenien* (Leipzig: Deuticke, 1911), chap. V, 56–57. English version: *Demenia Praecox or the Group of Schizophrenias* (New York: International Universities Press, 1950).
4. Karolinska Institute. The Nobel Prize in Physiology or Medicine, 2000. http://noble.prize.org
5. Arthur Schopenhauer, *The World as Will and Idea*, 1818, ii, 199: Essays, "On Noise." Translated by Will Durant, *The Story of Philosophy* (New York: Simon and Schuster, 1953), 230.

6. Sigmund Freud, "The Case of Schreber," vol. XII, *The Standard Edition of the Complete Psychological Works of Sigmund Freud*, trans. James Strachey (London: The Hogarth Press, 1958), 90.
7. Harry Stack Sullivan, *Schizophrenia as a Human Process* (New York: WW Norton and Company, 1962), 243–244; the remarks were comments following a speech he made after delivering a paper published in 1931.
8. Jean Delay and Pierre Deniker (1952), trans. Murray Jarvik, 166. L. S. Goodman and A. Gilman, *The Pharmacological Basis of Therapeutics* (New York: Macmillan, 1965).
9. Paul E. Meehl, "Schizotaxia, Schizotypy, Schizophrenia," *American Psychologist* 17, no. 12 (1962): 827–838.
10. Bishop George Berkeley, *Treatise Concerning the Principles of Human Knowledge* (Dublin: Jeremy Pepyat, 1710), 22–23; http://plato.stanford.edu/entries/berkeley.
11. Plato, *The Republic*, trans. Benjamin Jowett (New York: The Colonial Press, 1901), http://ww.fordham.edu/halsall/ancient/plato-republic.txt.

Chapter 2

1. E. Robins and S. B. Guze, "Establishment of Diagnostic Validity in Psychiatric Illness: Its Application to Schizophrenia," *American Journal of Psychiatry* 126 (1970), 983–987.
2. Donald Broadbent, *Perception and Communication* (Oxford, England: Pergamon, 1958).
3. P. H. Venables, "Input Dysfunction in Schizophrenia," *Progress in Experimental Personality Research* 72 (1964): 1–47.
4. D. Hawkins and L. Pauling, *Orthmolecular Psychiatry: Treatment of Schizophrenia* (San Francisco: W. H. Freeman and Co., 1973).
5. P. G. Zimbardo, S. M. Andersen, and L. G. Kabat, "Induced Hearing Deficit Generates Experimental Paranoia," *Science* 212 (1981): 1529–1531.
6. R. Freedman, M. Waldo, P. Bickford-Wimer, and H. Nagamoto, "Elementary Neuronal Dysfunctions in Schizophrenia," *Schizophrenia Research* 4 (1991): 233–243.

Chapter 3

1. J. C. Eccles, *The Inhibitory Pathways of the Central Nervous System* (Liverpool, England: Liverpool University Press, 1969).
2. R. Freedman, L. E. Adler, P. Bickford, W. Byerley, H. Coon, M. C. Cullum, J. M. Griffith, J. G. Harris, S. Leonard, C. Miller, M. Myles-Worsley, H. T. Nagamoto, G. M. Rose, and M. Waldo, "Schizophrenia and Nicotinic Receptors," *Harvard Review of Psychiatry* 2 (1994): 179–192.

Chapter 4

1. R. Freedman, C. Wetmore, I. Stromberg, S. Leonard, and L. Olson, "Alpha-Bungarotoxin Binding to Hippocampal Interneurons: Immunocytochemical Characterization and Effects on Growth Factor Expression," *Journal of Neuroscience* 13 (1993): 1965–1975.
2. Bernard Katz, *Nerve, Muscle, and Synapse* (Blacklick, Ohio: McGraw-Hill, 1966).

Chapter 5

1. S. S. Kety, D. Rosenthal, P. H. Wender, and F. Schulsinger, "Mental Illness in the Biological and Adoptive Families of Adopted Schizophrenics," *American Journal of Psychiatry* 128 (1971): 302–311.
2. R. Freedman, H. Coon, M. Myles-Worsley, A. Orr-Urtreger, A. Olincy, A. Davis, M. Polymeropoulos, J. Holik, J. Hopkins, M. Hoff, et al. "Linkage of a Neurophysiological Deficit in Schizophrenia to a Chromosome 15 Locus," *Proceedings of the National Academy of Sciences* 94 (1997): 587–592.
3. H. Stefansson, D. Rujescu, S. Cichon, A. Ingason, S. Steinberg, R. Fossdal, E. Sigurdsson, T. Sigmundsson, J. E. Buizer-Voskamp, T. Hansen, et al. "Large Recurrent Microdeletions Associated with Schizophrenia," *Nature* 455 (2008): 232–236.
4. J. Stone for the International Schizophrenia Consortium, "Rare Chromosomal Deletions and Duplications Increase Risk of Schizophrenia," *Nature* 455 (2008): 237–241.

Chapter 6

1. Jonathan Edwards, *Sinners in the Hands of an Angry God* (New Kingston, PA: Whitaker House, 1997).
2. H. S. Sullivan, *Schizophrenia as a Human Process* (New York: W. W. Norton, 1962).
3. Sylvia Nasar, *A Beautiful Mind: A Biography of John Forbes Nash, Jr., Winner of the Nobel Prize in Economics* (New York: Simon & Schuster, 1998).
4. W. A. Falls, M. J. Miserendino, and M. Davis, "Extinction of Fear-Potentiated Startle: Blockade by Infusion of an NMDA Antagonist into the Amygdala," *Journal of Neuroscience* 12 (1992): 854–863.
5. D. C. Javitt and S. R. Zukin, "Recent Advances in the Phencyclidine Model of Schizophrenia," *American Journal of Psychiatry* 148 (1991): 1301–1308.

6. G. Marsicano, C. T. Wotjak, S. C. Azad, T. Bisogno, G. Rammes, M. G. Cascio, H. Hermann, J. Tang, C. Hofmann, W. Zieglgansberger, M. V. Di, and B. Lutz, "The Endogenous Cannabinoid System Controls Extinction of Aversive Memories," *Nature* 418 (2002): 530–534.

Chapter 7

1. M. F. Green, "What are the Functional Consequences of Neurocognitive Deficits in Schizophrenia," *American Journal of Psychiatry* 153 (1996): 321–330.
2. G. E. Hogarty, N. R. Schooler, R. Ulrich, F. Mussare, P. Ferro, and E. Herron, "Fluphenazine and Social Therapy in the Aftercare of Schizophrenic Patients: Relapse Analyses of a Two-Year Controlled Study of Fluphenazine Decanoate and Fluphenazine Hydrochloride," *Archives of General Psychiatry* 36 (1979): 1283–1294.
3. Richard Warner, *Recovery from Schizophrenia: Psychiatry and Political Economy,* 3rd edition (New York: Psychology Press, 2004).
4. Elliot S. Valentstein, *Brain Control: A Critical Examination of Brain Stimulation and Psychosurgery* (New York: Wiley, 1973).
5. C. M. Harding, G. W. Brooks, T. Ashikaga, J. S. Strauss, and A. Breier, "The Vermont Longitudinal Study of Persons with Severe Mental Illness, II: Long-Term Outcome of Subjects Who Retrospectively Met DSM-III Criteria for Schizophrenia," *American Journal of Psychiatry* 144 (1987): 727–735.
6. P. R. May, A. H. Tuma, W. J. Dixon, C. Yale, D. A. Thiele, and W. H. Kraude, "Schizophrenia: A Follow-Up Study of the Results of Five Forms of Treatment," *Archives of General Psychiatry* 38, no. 7 (1981): 776–784.
7. Jean Delay and Pierre Deniker (1952), translated by Murray Jarvik, in L. S. Goodman and A. Gilman, *The Pharmacological Basis of Therapeutics* (New York: Macmillan, 1965), 166.
8. Solomon H. Snyder, *Drugs, Madness, and the Brain* (London: Hart-Davis, MacGibbon, Ltd. 1975).

Chapter 8

1. J. Kane, G. Honigfeld, J. Singer, and H. Meltzer, "Clozapine for the Treatment-Resistant Schizophrenic: A Double-Blind Comparison with Chlorpromazine," *Archives of General Psychiatry* 45 (1988): 789–796.
2. J. A. Lieberman, T. S. Stroup, J. P. McEvoy, M. S. Swartz, R. A. Rosenheck, D. O. Perkins, R. S. Keefe, S. M. Davis, C. E. Davis, B. D. Lebowitz, et al., "Clinical Antipsychotic Trials of Intervention

Effectiveness (CATIE) Investigators: Effectiveness of Antipsychotic Drugs in Patients with Chronic Schizophrenia," *New England Journal of Medicine* 353 (2005): 1209–1223.

3. T. P. George, M. J. Sernyak, D. M. Ziedonis, and S. W. Woods, "Effects of Clozapine on Smoking in Chronic Schizophrenic Outpatients," *Journal of Clinical Psychiatry* 56 (1995): 344–346.

4. A. Olincy, J. G. Harris, L. L. Johnson, V. Pender, S. Kongs, D. Allensworth, J. Ellis, G. O. Zerbe, S. Leonard, K. E. Stevens, et al., "Proof-of-Concept Trial of an α7-Nicotinic Agonist in Schizophrenia," *Archives of General Psychiatry* 63 (2006): 630–638.

Chapter 9

1. R. Freedman, R. Ross, R. Michels, P. Appelbaum, L. Siever, R. Binder, W. Carpenter, S. H. Friedman, P. Resnick, and J. Rosenbaum, "Psychiatrists, Mental Illness, and Violence," *American Journal of Psychiatry* 164 (2007): 1315–1317.

2. J. Leff, N. N. Wig, H. Bedi, D. K. Menon, L. Kuipers, A. Korten, G. Ernberg, R. Day, N. Sartorius, and A. Jablensky, "Relatives' Expressed Emotion and the Course of Schizophrenia in Chandigarh: A Two-Year Follow-up of a First-Contact Sample," *British Journal of Psychiatry* 156 (1990): 351–356.

Chapter 10

1. J. A. Court, S. Lloyd, M. Johnson, M. Griffiths, N. J. M. Birdsall, M. A. Piggott, A. E. Oakley, P. G. Ince, E. K. Perry, and R. H. Perry, "Nicotinic and Muscarinic Cholinergic Receptor Binding in the Human Hippocampal Formation during Development and Aging," *Developmental Brain Research* 101 (1997): 93–105.

2. C. E. Adams, J. A. Stitzel, A. C. Collins, and R. Freedman, "Alpha7-Nicotinic Receptor Expression and the Anatomical Organization of Hippocampal Interneurons," *Brain Research* 922 (2001): 180–190.

3. M. Alkondon, E. F. R. Pereira, W. S. Cortes, A. Maelicke, and E. X. Albuquerque, "Choline Is a Selective Agonist at Alpha7 Nicotinic Acetylcholine Receptors in Rat Brain Neurons," *European Journal of Neuroscience* 9 (1997): 2734–2742.

4. R. Freedman, M. Hall, L. E. Adler, and S. Leonard, "Evidence in Postmortem Brain Tissue for Decreased Numbers of Hippocampal Nicotinic Receptors in Schizophrenia," *Biological Psychiatry* 38 (1995): 22–33.

5. R. H. Porter, S. L. Eastwood, and P. J. Harrison, "Distribution of Kainate Receptor Subunit mRNAs in Human Hippocampus, Neocortex and Cerebellum, and Bilateral Reduction of Hippocampal GluR6 and KA2 Transcripts in Schizophrenia," *Brain Research* 751 (1997): 217–231.
6. V. B. Aramakis, C. Y. Hsieh, F. M. Leslie, and R. Metherate, "A Critical Period for Nicotine-Induced Disruption of Synaptic Development in Rat Auditory Cortex," *Journal of Neuroscience* 20 (2000): 6106–6116.
7. S. H. Zeisel, "The Fetal Origins of Memory: The Role of Dietary Choline in Optimal Brain Development," *The Journal of Pediatrics* 149 (2006): S131–S136.
8. I. Melle, J. Olav, S. Friis, U. Haahr, I. Joa, T. K. Larsen, S. Opjordsmoen, B. R. Rund, E. Simonsen, P. Vaglum, and T. McGlashan, "Early Detection of the First Episode of Schizophrenia and Suicidal Behavior," *American Journal of Psychiatry* 163 (2006): 800–804.

Chapter 11

1. M. E. Scheibel and A. B. Scheibel, "Specialized Organizational Patterns within the Nucleus Reticularis Thalami of the Cat," *Experimental Neurology* 34 (1972): 316–322.
2. J. Court, D. Spurden, S. Lloyd, I. McKeith, C. Ballard, N. Cairns, R. Kerwin, R. Perry, and E. Perry, "Neuronal Nicotinic Receptors in Dementia with Lewy Bodies and Schizophrenia: Alpha-Bungarotoxin and Nicotine Binding in the Thalamus," *Journal of Neurochemistry* 73 (1999): 1590–1597.

Index

Note: All illustrations are indicated by page numbers in *italics*